Men'sHealth®

THE
BODY
YOU WANT
IN THE
TIME
YOU HAVE

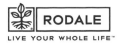

RODALE

LIVE YOUR WHOLE LIFE™

Every day our brands connect with and inspire millions of people to live a life of the mind, body, spirit — a whole life.

Men'sHealth.

THE
BODY
YOU WANT
IN THE
TIME
YOU HAVE

The Ultimate Guide to
Getting Leaner and Building
Stronger Muscles with
Workouts That Fit Any Schedule

MYATT MURPHY

RODALE

Notice

Photographs by Mitch Mandel/Rodale Images

Book design by Patricia Field

Library of Congress Cataloging-in-Publication Data

Murphy, Myatt.
    The body you want in the time you have : the ultimate guide to getting leaner and building stronger muscles with workouts that fit any schedule / Myatt Murphy.
        p.   cm.
    Includes index.
    ISBN-13 978—1—59486—242—7 hardcover
    ISBN-10 1—59486—242—7 hardcover
    ISBN-13 978—1—59486—243—4 paperback
    ISBN-10 1—59486—243—5 paperback
    1. Bodybuilding. 2. Exercise. 3. Time management. I. Title.
  GV546.5.M85 2005
  613.7'13—dc22   2005016472

Distributed to the trade by Holtzbrinck Publishers

4 6 8 10 9 7 5   hardcover

2 4 6 8 10 9 7 5 3   paperback

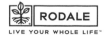

To my dad, whose exercise advice
changed my life and guided me on the
path of doing the same for millions of
men and women worldwide.
If this book gets you into great shape,
he's the one to thank.

Contents

Acknowledgments ix

Chapter 1: Time Is Muscle 1

Chapter 2: What Workout Do YOU Have Time For? 5

Chapter 3: All You Need to Know . . . And Nothing More! 15

Chapter 4: Your 48 "Anytime" Exercises 43

Chapter 5: I Have Only 1 Day a Week 143

Chapter 6: I Have Only 2 Days a Week 157

Chapter 7: I Have Only 3 Days a Week 177

Chapter 8: I Have 4 Days a Week 199

Chapter 9: I Have 5 Days a Week 229

Chapter 10: I Have 6 Days a Week 261

Chapter 11: I Have 7 Days a Week 295

Chapter 12: Your Minute-Man Nutrition Plan 307

Index 319

Acknowledgments

I want to truly thank the two editors to whom, over time, I realized I owe my career in magazines: Steve Perrine, who pushed me to develop a writing style, helped me find my voice, and taught me everything I know and still use today; and David Zinczenko, who pushed me harder than I would ever have pushed myself. Thank you both for bringing me back home to *Men's Health*. It feels good to come back and once again be a part of what started it all.

I also want to thank all the editors who have allowed me to share my quirky spin on exercise and fitness with millions of people for more than a decade now. I've had the pleasure of working with some of the best in the business, which is probably why I still enjoy what I do for a living. I hope that I haven't forgotten anyone on this list—but here it goes: Rochelle Udell, Lucy Danziger, Gabrielle Studenmund, Stephen George, Bobby Lee, Mike Carlson, Pamela Miller, Laura Gilbert, Jeff Csatari, Rosie Amodio, Duane Swierczynski, Ed Dwyer, Liz O'Brian, Jennifer Walters, Nicole Dorsey, Albert Baime, Alex Strauss, Beth Bischoff, Gordon Bass, Emily Spilko, Denise Brodey, Stephanie Young, Scott Quill, Nichele Hoskins, Mary Christ, Su Reid, Gail O'Connor, Abigail Walch, Dana Points, Lisa Delany, David Kalmansohn, Jerry Kindela, Nina Willdorf, and Alison Ashton.

A very special thanks to my assistant, Jon Addison, for putting in so many hours on this project—and the many projects before this one—and to the hundreds of exercise physiologists, personal trainers, and sports psychologists I've studied under, interviewed, trained with, and ghostwritten for. I've been fortunate to work with nearly every top fitness professional in the business, and there's no greater education than that.

Finally, I'd like to thank the three unwanted friends I made in 2004: Frances, Ivan, and Jeanne. Because of a schedule rush, I needed to write this book in exactly 40 days. Then, a combination of Hurricane Frances, Hurricane Ivan, and Hurricane Jeanne left my family homeless in Florida, left me officeless for a week, and swept my car downstream into another state. This book was written during three flood-producing hurricanes—and was still produced in 40 days. I won't touch upon the irony, but it proves that finding time—in the most ridiculous of circumstances—is always a possibility.

In other words, if I could find the time to write this book, then *you* can always find just a little time to exercise.

Time Is Muscle

Twenty to 30 minutes a day. Three times a week.

Sounds painfully familiar, doesn't it?

Whether you're new to exercise or are an exercise veteran who has long since paid your dues, you already know this tried-and-true fitness formula. It's every exercise expert's basic prescription for building the perfect physique. It's the underpinning program that guarantees to bring you the results your body has been waiting for. There's only one problem. If it's such a no-fail way to build muscle, burn fat, and stay fit . . .

. . . then why can't you seem to stick with it?

As *Men's Health* magazine's first fitness editor, it was my job to create as many inventive workouts as possible to motivate millions of readers to exercise on a monthly basis. With each article, I knew there was someone on the other end of those words who was being introduced to exercise for the very first time.

Since those days, I've had the pleasure of sharing my creative exercise knowledge through hundreds of workouts for more than 40 international magazines. Ten years and more than 100 million satisfied readers later, I've finally come to realize something I should have seen coming.

What if you have 20 to 30 minutes to spare, but you don't have 3 days a week? What if you have 3 days a week to exercise, but you can't give me 20 to 30 minutes? Or worse yet . . .

. . . what if you don't have either?

Not Enough Time

Life doesn't always play fair when it comes to making exercise convenient, does it? One minute, you have every intention of exercising for a half-hour. Then, somewhere between playing hide-and-seek with your car keys and having your boss decide you need to know about his recurring psoriasis, life suddenly leaves you debating whether it's worth changing your shorts for the 10-minute window you now have left to work out.

Even if you manage to find 30 minutes on one day to exercise, it doesn't mean that the rest of your week is going to be as kind. Life has a way of fast-pitching us curveballs that leave us with fewer days per week to spare. Suddenly, that

3-day-a-week promise you made to your muscles becomes a 1-day raincheck your body can't cash until the following week—if you're lucky.

Not Enough Results

Or is this you? Are you on the opposite side of the coin? Pushing the classic 3-day-a-week plan aside isn't always about having enough time to exercise. If mustering up enough minutes or staying dedicated to working out isn't your problem, maybe it's continuing to see the results you once did—or pushing toward the goals you still have for yourself—that's the real issue.

You probably remember the first time you starting seeing results from your exercise routine. Unfortunately, and inevitably, there comes a time when that basic 3-day-a-week fitness plan that once worked miracles to reshape your body will stop doing the trick. Exercise experts call it reaching a plateau, or hitting the wall, and it's the number one reason why most people give up on fitness all together. If you're not new to working out, then you know this place all too well. If you're just starting out, well, I'm afraid it's what you have to look forward to.

Or maybe not.

Not a Problem

I've got some news I think you and your body are really going to like. The truth is, it really doesn't matter that you can't exercise 3 days a week.

The only thing that matters *is that you exercise.*

You see, no matter how much time you can devote to working out, or how much exercise experience you have, you and everyone else reading this book pretty much want the same thing: more muscle and less fat.

Well, guess what?

No matter what level you're at with exercise, no matter what your personal goals are, no matter how much time you have for working out, no matter how many days a week you have to exercise, *this book is about to become your exercise guide for the rest of your life.*

Why? Because it's the first book that finally lets *you* call the shots when it comes to your workouts. All you need to know are the answers to three easy questions.

⊠ How many days can you exercise this week?

⊠ How much time can you work out each day?

⊠ What are your fitness goals?

After that, I'll do the rest.

With this book, you'll not only learn how to start exercising right now, but you'll also learn how to instantly adjust your workouts anytime—every single week of your life—without ever having to sacrifice the results you expect. In fact, you're going to build even stronger, leaner muscles because of it.

This book is organized according to time instead of expertise, so anyone—the beginner, the

NO MATTER WHAT LEVEL YOU'RE AT WITH EXERCISE, NO MATTER WHAT YOUR PERSONAL GOALS ARE, NO MATTER HOW MUCH TIME YOU HAVE FOR WORKING OUT, NO MATTER HOW MANY DAYS A WEEK YOU HAVE TO EXERCISE, *THIS BOOK IS ABOUT TO BECOME YOUR EXERCISE GUIDE FOR THE REST OF YOUR LIFE.*

intermediate exerciser, or the advanced athlete—can use it for maximum results. I don't care whether you have 10, 20, 30, or 60 minutes to hit the weights. I don't care whether you can exercise only 1 or 2 days a week, whether you have time to do the 3 or 4 days a week that most experts recommend, or whether you're ready to push yourself to new heights by trying a 5-, 6-, or 7-day workout schedule.

From this day forward, time is no longer a factor when it comes to interfering with your exercise plans. Each and every chapter delivers its own perfect workout for the amount of time given. Now, the next time life either shortchanges you for time or gives you more than you expected, you'll be ready to utilize the time you *do* have to your greatest advantage!

Are you looking to take your body one step further . . . without having to try any harder? It's easy when you have the right diet working side by side with your workouts. That's why I've created the Minute-Man Nutrition Plan, the eating strategy in chapter 12 that works like everything else in this book. Do you have only 4 minutes a day to think about eating healthy? 3? 2? Oh, don't tell me you have only 1! Even if that's the case, it's okay, because once you know the 12 easiest tweaks for healthy eating, you can tailor your diet in seconds to ensure that you always get the absolute best nutrition for your body . . . in the least amount of time!

With this combination of diet and exercise, I've written you the perfect prescription to get in shape. Only now, I'm making sure that you can fill that prescription every day of the week, every week of the year, and every year of your life—no matter what life decides to throw at you.

If you're ready to learn how to get in shape in any situation, I've got time for you.

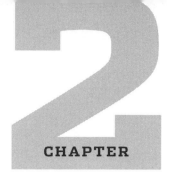

What Workout Do YOU Have Time For?

Why Anything Is Always Better Than Nothing

When it comes to exercise, there's a simple two-word phrase I never, ever want you to forget: Everything counts.

For the majority of you reading this book, working out 3 days a week may seem like a goal that's well beyond your reach. But just because you don't have much time to exercise, that doesn't necessarily mean that it's not worth making an effort.

ANY EXERCISE IS AN INVESTMENT

Not exercising because you have only a few minutes is like never bothering to put money in the bank because all you have are a few pennies to throw in. Sure, you have high hopes about the amount of cash you would like to see in your bank account. And yes, the more money you can part with each week, the faster you'll hit that total. But if you can never manage to save anything, your odds of *ever* saving even when you finally have extra money are next to none. Likewise, if you can part with a few pennies a week, you'll be that much closer to making that grand total a reality one day.

The same theory applies to exercise. I'm not going to lie to you: Not having as much time to exercise does mean that it may take you longer to see the results you're gunning for. But doing anything—even if all you have in you is 10 minutes a week—will bring you one small step closer to realizing your goals. It also means you won't have to work as hard once you finally have a few more minutes—or days—to exercise.

A LITTLE EXERCISE CAN KEEP YOUR MUSCLES GUESSING

If you're an intermediate or advanced exerciser—or even if you're a beginner who's managed to exercise for a few weeks without quitting—having life shorten your workouts once in a while may be just what you need for seeing better results. You see, muscles adapt to any exercise routine quickly, adjusting themselves within six to eight workouts. After that, your body learns to perform whatever workout you're doing by using less effort. Where does that leave your body? Well, it makes each time you exercise *less* effective for building muscle, burning fat, or improving your cardiovascular health.

Having to do a shorter workout because you're pressed for time forces you to try new routines. It forces you to use different exercises that can keep your muscles challenged enough to continue growing and improving.

A LITTLE EXERCISE MAKES YOU MORE RESILIENT TO INJURIES

Lack of time may even help keep you exercising injury-free. Your body isn't much different from a set of tires on your car. Fail to rotate your tires every once in a while and you'll pay for it by wearing them out a lot faster in certain spots.

Sticking with the same exercise routine can have the same effect on your body, causing specific joints, tendons, and tissues to wear down from overuse. When time interferes with your workout plans, adjusting with a shorter routine every so often can prevent all that unnecessary wear and tear by giving certain overused areas a break.

A LITTLE EXERCISE INCREASES YOUR FITNESS EDUCATION

The average exerciser relies on the same handful of exercises in his personal workout repertoire. When life throws a monkey wrench in your workout schedule, you can use it as an opportunity to work on your exercise education—a degree that most exercisers never bother to earn. Time crunches can give you the chance to try exercises, machines, and workouts you may otherwise never have bothered to learn. The more that life messes with your plans, the more diverse types of exercises you'll have to try, which exposes your body to new challenges for even greater results—that is, if you know what adjustments to make to your workout. But don't worry; that's what this book is all about.

A LITTLE EXERCISE IS PROBABLY ALL YOU WOULD DO ANYWAY, EVEN IF YOU HAD MORE TIME

Most people spend more time in the gym than they have to, lengthening their workouts in ways that can actually be counterproductive to their goals. If you think about it, are you really *exercising* throughout the entire length of a workout? Of course not! Sure, you could devote a full hour to exercise, but that wouldn't mean you'd actually spend a full hour doing it. Remove all the typical social distractions (reading, watching TV, chatting up anything blonde, sweaty, and Swedish) and the time most people truly spend

THE MORE THAT LIFE MESSES WITH YOUR PLANS, THE MORE DIVERSE TYPES OF EXERCISES YOU'LL HAVE TO TRY, WHICH EXPOSES YOUR BODY TO NEW CHALLENGES FOR EVEN GREATER RESULTS—THAT IS, IF YOU KNOW WHAT ADJUSTMENTS TO MAKE TO YOUR WORKOUT.

exercising can boil down to less than 20 minutes a workout.

Doing your routine in a time-efficient way can be a healthier decision in the long run. Cutting corners in a routine can have its own set of health benefits—if you know which corners to cut.

- ☒ Waiting less time between exercises can make your weight-lifting routine more aerobic in nature, which can help you burn more calories and fat as a side perk.

- ☒ Doing only 1 set of an exercise instead of a few can exhaust your muscles just as effectively, especially since many people give their all only on the last set of every exercise.

- ☒ Picking exercises that work more muscle groups in one shot can teach your muscles to work together, making them function better during other activities, sports, and everyday tasks.

SO YOU HAVE ONLY 20 MINUTES OR LESS TO GIVE ME?

So what?

If 10 to 20 minutes is all you can spare, then you already have more than enough time to give your body what it desperately needs. The next time you're forced to give me the bare minimum of minutes, keep the following thoughts in mind so your muscles don't feel guilty.

Your muscles aren't as lazy as you think. Most people wait too long between exercises, giving their muscles unnecessary time to cool down. Creatine phosphate, the fuel your muscles use for anaerobic activity, returns within 30 seconds to 2 minutes, depending on the intensity of your exercise regime. Resting that long doesn't make your body any stronger; it just makes your workouts longer.

Your body burns fat no matter how long you exercise. Your body turns to two main sources whenever it needs fuel for energy: glycogen (carbohydrates stored within your muscles) and your own body fat. Although your heart rate does need to be elevated for at least 20 minutes before your body needs to dip into its fat stores for energy, you're still burning excess calories whether you work out for 1 minute or 1 hour. Even if your body burns mostly calories from stored carbohydrates, you'll have fewer in your system for your body to assume you need to store as fat.

Your routine may not need as many sets as you think. Having time to do only 1 set of an exercise isn't better for your body, but it's not bad for it either, as long as you perform that exercise at a high intensity. Researchers at the University of Florida had subjects perform 1 set of an exercise at a high intensity, while another group performed 3 sets of the same exercise at a low intensity. After 14 weeks, both groups showed nearly the same results in muscle growth. The reason? One theory is that most people save their strength for their 3rd set, making the first 2 sets nothing more than a warmup. So, as long as you make the 1st set of every exercise count, doing just that 1 set is still enough to build muscle.

Your brain may need less to think about. Doing three or four exercises per muscle group can be very effective at promoting more muscular growth, but only if you're making your muscles work throughout your entire workout. Having too many exercises to choose from can cause less-motivated individuals to reserve their efforts just to make it through their lengthy, self-imposed workouts. Simplifying your workout to one exercise per muscle group can help bring back that intensity, letting you push yourself as hard as possible for maximum muscle fatigue.

The Workout You're *Supposed* to Have Time For!

Here it is: the workout that most experts agree is the best launching point for exercise, regardless of what you look like now—or what you plan on looking like later. It really doesn't matter what type of physique you're hoping to develop in the future. It typically starts with this 3-day-a-week, 20-to-30-minutes a day, basic eight-move exercise plan.

MONDAY, WEDNESDAY, AND FRIDAY

Do 3 sets of 8 to 12 repetitions except where noted.

Squat

Lunge

Bench press

One-arm row

Seated shoulder press

Seated triceps extension

Biceps curl

Crunch (3 sets of 12 to 15 repetitions)

If you're not familiar with these exercises yet—or maybe need a little reminder of how to do them properly—just turn to chapter 4 and introduce yourself to them. Otherwise, don't worry. Right now, all I want to do is educate you in the basics or remind you why you should still know them by heart.

SO WHY IS THIS PLAN THE BEST TO START WITH?

Good question. Many people who've been using this plan for years probably couldn't give you a definitive answer to that. But there's a reason this eight-move routine—or variations on the same principle—continues to stand the test of time. In fact, there are a whole bunch of reasons why this plan is the best basic program for exercisers of all levels.

IT LEAVES NO STONE UNTURNED

Each of the eight exercises in the basic plan targets a specific muscle group.

- The squat works your legs (from your butt to your calves).
- The lunge also works your legs (from your butt to your calves).
- The bench press works your chest, shoulders, and triceps (the back of your arms).
- The one-arm row works your upper and lower back.
- The seated shoulder press works your shoulders.
- The seated triceps extension works your triceps.
- The biceps curl works your biceps (the front of your arms).
- The crunch works your abdominals.

When combined, these moves form a full-body routine that acts as exercise insurance for your muscles, making sure that you never forget to challenge any of them by accident.

Why does that matter?

Well, most people exercise with a few body parts already in mind—typically, the ones they want to change. Maybe your goal is to pack on a bigger, stronger chest or to trim down to a tighter waistline. Maybe it's to build sleeve-ripping biceps or simply to have a lean, chiseled look that makes the statue of David envious of your muscular definition.

Since most people tend to tailor their workouts to whichever body part needs immediate improvement, they may easily abandon the basics and stray from achieving a total body balance.

Lofty goals of big arms or a better butt usually make the average exerciser ignore other muscles that are critical for creating full-body symmetry. This can keep you from a more impressive physique, since the muscles you may be ignoring may also be important to exercise to help develop the areas you really want to reshape. Keeping the body in balance allows your muscles to work together instead of resisting each other. The basic eight-move workout plan makes sure all your major muscle groups work equally for a complete, balanced look.

IT'S MADE UP OF THE MOST-EFFECTIVE MOVES

This average beginner's program uses mostly compound exercises—exercises in which several muscles work together—instead of isolation exercises, which target just one specific muscle group. For example, to do the chest press with the proper form, your chest, shoulder, and triceps muscles all have to pitch in. These types of compound exercises are far more practical for building lean muscle fast, because they work more muscle fibers in a shorter period of time. They're also effective in teaching your body to function more efficiently, since they help train your muscles to work more thoroughly and efficiently with each other.

IT'S IN THE PERFECT ORDER

Choosing which muscles to exercise first is like picking a good team in gym class. Start with the smaller, lanky nerds and your team has a snowball's chance in hell of pulling out a win. You want to pick the biggest teammates (and similarly the biggest muscle groups) first, with good reason. The multijoint exercises used to work large muscle groups, such as the squat or any pressing movements, always require smaller muscles to help stabilize the body. Tire those tiny muscles first and they'll quit on you before you get a chance to exhaust the larger muscles enough to make them improve.

The best exercise programs are always designed to work larger muscle groups (legs, back, and chest) first and smaller muscle groups (shoulders, triceps, biceps, calves, and abs) last.

IT'S THE PERFECT RECIPE FOR RESULTS

Quick lesson: A *repetition* is simply an exercise performed one time (both lifting and lowering the

> LOFTY GOALS OF BIG ARMS OR A BETTER BUTT USUALLY MAKE THE AVERAGE EXERCISER IGNORE OTHER MUSCLES THAT ARE CRITICAL FOR CREATING FULL-BODY SYMMETRY. THIS CAN KEEP YOU FROM A MORE IMPRESSIVE PHYSIQUE.

weight). A *set* is a group of repetitions. Doing 1 set of 8 to 12 repetitions means performing the exercise 8 to 12 times. Now that you know that, here's why the basic eight-move plan is considered the ideal starting point.

Experts consider doing 3 sets of an exercise before moving on to the next exercise the magic number for the greatest amount of overall muscular development. The basic plan also limits the amount of repetitions you should do for each exercise to 8 to 12. This is also considered to be the ideal number for anyone looking for a stronger, firmer, leaner physique.

Using a weight you can heave only six to eight times builds more muscular size and power, creating a larger, stronger physique but one that's less well-defined. Choosing a weight you can lift 12 to 15 times will improve muscular endurance, leaving you with a leaner look—especially when mixed with aerobic exercise—but less size in your muscles. Sticking with 8 to 12 repetitions per exercise is considered the best of all worlds, since it helps you build quality muscle that's just the right size.

IT GIVES YOUR MUSCLES ALL THE REST THEY NEED

The basic eight-move plan schedules your 3-day workouts every other day (Monday, Wednesday, and Friday, for example). Why is this perfect? Because it leaves just enough time for muscles to recuperate and rebuild from exercise.

Your muscles don't actually grow when you're sweating in the weight room; they grow while you're sleeping in bed. Weight lifting causes microscopic tears within the muscle fibers that need time to repair themselves. Muscles grow best when they're given at least 48 hours of rest. Giving a muscle less time than that doesn't allow the fibers to rebuild themselves, whereas too much rest doesn't keep them challenged enough to bother. The 3-day-a-week plan makes sure that you always get just enough rest between your workouts—never more, and never less.

IT KEEPS YOU INJURY-FREE

As I already mentioned, starting yourself on a full-body routine early will ensure that you'll have a strong, symmetrical build. But having a balanced body isn't important just for looking good, it's also critical when it comes to feeling good. The injuries that pull even the most devout exerciser away from his routine are almost always the result of forgetting this simple rule of muscular equality. Repetitive-use injuries (such as tennis elbow and

shin splints) and sudden muscle sprains or strains are usually the result of a muscular imbalance that could easily have been prevented.

All it takes to prevent these causes of injury is to remember *all* your muscles when you exercise. The basic eight-move plan gets you in that habit right from the start.

Why Your Body Should Never Settle For the Basics

Exercising just 20 to 30 minutes a day, three times a week, is a great starting point for getting fit. But if you never push yourself any harder than that, you may end up holding your muscles back. Maybe you're already at a level of fitness where 3 days a week, 20 to 30 minutes a day isn't enough to see results. (If you're not there yet, you will be soon, using the programs in this book!) When you finally *do* have more time to give, your body will reward you with even more results.

YOU'LL BURN MORE CALORIES—AND BODY FAT!

As explained earlier, whenever your body needs fuel for energy, it turns to two main sources: glycogen (carbohydrates stored within your muscles) and your own body fat. For the first 20 minutes of your workout, your body relies mostly on glycogen for energy. The good news is that your body can store only so much glycogen. After your glycogen stores run out—after 20 minutes or so—your body is left with no choice as you continue your workout but to burn body fat.

YOU CAN ADD MORE VARIETY TO YOUR WORKOUTS

Eventually, your muscles get used to whatever program you're using on them. That boredom can lead to a *plateau*—which is when your body stops

THE RESULTS YOUR BODY ALWAYS HAS TIME FOR!

Whether life leaves you with a little time to exercise or a lot, your body is guaranteed to benefit from your efforts. Here's a rundown of the results you can expect if you follow the guidelines I'm going to teach you.

What You Can Do	What You'll Get Back!
10 min per workout	An intense workout that maximizes convenience and minimizes wear and tear on your joints, tendons, and bones
20 min per workout	A time-efficient, intense workout with little wear and tear; its duration is at the lower end of the recommended ideal range
30 min per workout	Time to add more exercises for more results; a duration at the higher end of the recommended ideal range
45 min per workout	More calorie-burning, muscle-building benefits than the average workout; more time to isolate individual muscle groups
60 min per workout	Maximum fat and calorie burn; time for the most-thorough exercise options
1 day per week	A perfect starting point for beginners; a maintenance plan that prevents intermediate and advanced exercisers from ever losing muscle
2 days per week	A workout that's 90 percent as effective at shaping muscle as exercising 3 days is!
3 days per week	The ideal prescription for results: more muscle with the least risk of overuse injury
4 days per week	The freedom to split up your routines; stronger muscles; the time to try more-unique exercises
5 days per week	More definition; more time to try advanced routines for even more-impressive results
6 or 7 days per week	The most variety in your workouts; the most time to focus on every muscle group individually for maximum results

showing results from your exercise routine. The longer you can make your workouts, the more exercises you can add to them, which brings even more possible variations for your muscles to grow from.

Being able to add more moves is also a plus for larger muscle groups such as your back, chest, shoulders, and legs. Smaller muscle groups (such as your biceps, triceps, and calves) need only one to three exercises to work them

thoroughly enough to help them improve. But larger muscle groups are typically made up of several separate muscles that work together. To work your back, legs, shoulders, and chest as thoroughly as your smaller muscles, you need to hit each of these muscles with two to four exercises—an intermediate option that extra time can give you. The more moves you can add into your program, the faster you'll see the results you're looking for.

YOU'LL HAVE TIME TO TARGET INDIVIDUAL MUSCLE GROUPS

For time's sake, many of the exercises used in shorter weight-lifting programs are multijoint movements that force several muscle groups to work together, letting you strengthen and shape all of them at the same time. However, to really target a particular muscle group, you need to use certain single-joint exercises that specifically isolate that muscle group by preventing other muscles from helping out.

Having the time to use more exercises in your program lets you keep the basic multijoint exercises you "have" to do, plus, at the intermediate level, add more single-range, isolation exercises that work whichever muscles you feel need more improvement. That means you'll have more opportunities to focus extra attention on whatever area you feel needs to get leaner, bigger, or stronger.

YOU'LL BUILD MUSCLE EVEN FASTER!

With less time, a full-body routine that works all of your muscles on the same day—3 days per week—is recommended.

If you have more than 3 days each week to exercise, you can take advantage of an intermediate to advanced training technique known as a *split*

routine. Instead of doing all your exercises in one routine, you can split your full-body routine into two sessions—or even into three sessions, if you have 6 days to exercise. Breaking up your routine lets you use even more exercises, so you can re-shape your muscles from almost every angle.

SO YOU HAVE MORE THAN 20 MINUTES TO GIVE ME?

Congratulations! You'll be happy to know that once you're able to improve upon the traditional 3-day-a-week, 20-to-30-minutes-a-day program, you'll reach your goals a lot faster than before. That is, if you know how to ease into all that extra time. The following rules will keep you from pushing yourself *too* hard.

Longer doesn't have to mean harder. If at any time during the week you begin to feel burned-out, overly sore, or fatigued from exercise, chances are you could be *overtraining*. Overtraining occurs when you've pushed your body to the point where it can't recover as well as usual from your workouts, and that can lead to fatigue, moodiness, persistent muscular soreness, sleep problems, loss of appetite, and a lack of desire to exercise. In addition to making you feel lousy, overtraining works against your fitness goals because your muscles stop improving and become more at risk for injury.

Not giving your muscles enough rest between sets, doing too many sets and/or exercises per muscle group, and exercising too often can all lead to overtraining. If you follow the routines in this book, you should be fine, since each gives your muscles the 48 hours they require to rebuild themselves before you exercise them again.

However, overtraining can sometimes depend on the individual. Exercising just 2 or 3 days a

> EXERCISING JUST 2 OR 3 DAYS A WEEK CAN BE TOO MUCH FOR SOME PEOPLE AT THE START, WHEREAS OTHERS MAY BE ABLE TO TRAIN 6 DAYS A WEEK WITHOUT A BREAK AND NEVER OVERDO IT.

week can be too much for some people at the start, whereas others may be able to train 6 days a week without a break and never overdo it. To keep an eye on your own body, whatever your workout schedule is, you can take your pulse every morning. If it ever rises higher than five beats above your normal average, you could be overtraining or getting sick. In either case, it's a smart idea to take it easy for a few days.

Longer doesn't always mean more exercises. When striving for more muscle size and strength, many people make the mistake of doing too many exercises per muscle group. That can fatigue your muscles to a point where they are unable to build themselves back up as quickly—which can cause diminished results or even lead to a strain, a tear, or another exercise-related injury.

Going beyond four exercises per muscle group may work for advanced bodybuilders, but that's because many professionals use performance-enhancing drugs such as steroids that enable their bodies to recover from this type of intensive exercise a lot faster. Sticking with one to three exercises for smaller muscle groups (such as your biceps, triceps, and calves) and two to four exercises for larger muscle groups (such as your chest, back, legs, shoulders, and abdominals) is your safest bet for maximum results with the least amount of risk.

CHAPTER 3

All You Need to Know . . . And Nothing More!

The Basics You'd Better Know Before You Start

If getting in shape is so complicated, then why are so many witless people in better shape than you are?

The answer is simple.

Every occupation has its trade secrets—those little nuggets of insider info that make life easier for the few who know them, while those who don't are left clueless, with nothing to show for their efforts.

Well, that's not going to be you.

Understanding the basic rules of exercise can help you see why the 3-day-a-week plan is the most widely prescribed program for a basic full-body routine. But more important, it can help you to easily change that classic plan around for even more results.

Ready to learn the only rules you need to know for building a body you can be proud of, without ever wasting more effort than you have to spend?

Here's all you need to know . . . and nothing more . . . about strength training.

STRENGTH TRAINING 101

If you think of your muscles with mathematics in mind, changing them to look like you want them to is a lot easier than most people realize. Once you decide how you want your muscles to look, it's really just a matter of using the right combinations of numbers: repetitions, sets, and the amount of weight you should use. Learning why these numbers are so important to strength training will help you understand every plan in this book, plus it'll help you stick to your workouts in the long run.

No matter what program you end up using each week, here's all you need to know to get the most from every single exercise.

BEFORE YOU LIFT A SINGLE WEIGHT . . .

Know your reps. If you're strength training for muscular size and power, the best plan is to lift the weight for 6 to 8 repetitions in each set. If you're strength training for muscular endurance and a leaner look, then doing 12 to 15 repetitions per set is considered the smartest play. If you're looking for the best of both worlds, meaning muscles that are both strong and lean, then 8 to 12 repetitions per set are the numbers you want to remember.

Know your load. You'll want to choose a weight—or any form of resistance—that lets you do an exercise for only the exact number of repetitions recommended in each plan (no more and no less).

Know your potential. You may be anxious to see results, but using more weight than you are ready to handle increases your risk of getting injured.

So when should you try to use more weight? For any exercise, increase the amount of weight only when you can lift *more than* the number of reps assigned for *all* the sets of that exercise. Once you can do that, increase the weight in small increments (adding approximately 5 percent of the weight you're already using) until you're able to do the exercise for only the required number of reps again.

Know whether you're ready. If you can afford the time, warming up your muscles with some form of light, low-intensity cardiovascular activity for a few minutes before you lift can help them get more from every exercise. When you raise the temperature of a muscle through light exercise, you decrease its risk of injury by making the muscle more pliable. This extra flexibility gives your muscles a greater range of motion, letting you activate more muscle fibers as you exercise, for more results.

Before each strength-training workout, be sure to warm up your muscles with 5 minutes of a low-intensity cardiovascular exercise. Cycling in a low gear, parking farther from your gym so that you have to walk a few minutes to get there, or simply walking in place in your basement all work just fine.

AS YOU STRENGTH-TRAIN . . .

Take a breath. Many people try to hold in their breath as they raise the weights, which only raises your blood pressure and prevents you from taking in enough oxygen. Your body and muscles desperately need oxygen for energy. Plus, the less oxygen your muscles have to draw from, the less effective they are at contracting, which can inhibit how much weight they can lift. Handling less weight than you should be able to lift can slow down your overall results, since your muscles never get as much of a stimulus to evoke them to change.

Keep a steady flow of air moving through your lungs as you raise and lower the weights, exhaling as you raise the weight and inhaling as you lower the weight.

Take a look ahead. Jerking your head like some cymbal-playing monkey to see who's watching you is the fastest way to hurt yourself. Almost every upper-body exercise requires the erector spinae (a set of muscles that run along the sides of your spine) to help stabilize the back as you lift. These muscles end within your neck, which means they stay in a semistate of contraction every time you exercise. Looking around is like pulling on a rubber band that's already stretched as far as it can go. Moving in any direction can cause soft tissue strain or can stress the disks within your spine.

Always look straight ahead as you exercise, keeping your neck in line with your back. If you need to watch your form, stand far enough from a mirror so that you can see what you're doing without having to turn your neck.

Take your time. For most people, exercise is a constant ritual of pushing or pulling a weight in a given direction, then letting gravity take over to lower the weight back down. However, lowering a weight is just as effective for changing the shape, strength, and size of a muscle as raising it is.

By maintaining a slower pace, you can make sure your muscles never miss out on getting both benefits from every exercise.

Going too fast as you raise or lower a weight also makes it easy to shift your body around as you lift. This lets momentum help cheat the weight up, preventing the muscles you're trying to hit from getting a full workout, while increasing your odds of injuring any secondary muscles or tendons that are indirectly being thrown into the movement. Taking it slow lets you isolate the muscles you're trying to work, without using any that shouldn't be working in the first place. It's a tactic that lets you reap more muscle-building results with less risk of injury.

FOR MOST PEOPLE, EXERCISE IS A CONSTANT RITUAL OF PUSHING OR PULLING A WEIGHT IN A GIVEN DIRECTION. HOWEVER, LOWERING A WEIGHT IS JUST AS EFFECTIVE FOR CHANGING THE SHAPE, STRENGTH, AND SIZE OF A MUSCLE AS RAISING IT IS.

Experts agree that the best pace is to raise the weight for 2 seconds and lower it for 2 seconds. Using that speed, it's easy to see how much time 1 set of an exercise actually takes up. For example, if you maintain this tempo, then:

- ☒ Every set that ranges from 6 to 8 repetitions should take approximately 24 to 32 seconds to complete—or an average of 28 seconds.

- ☒ Every set that ranges from 8 to 12 repetitions should take approximately 32 to 48 seconds to complete—or an average of 40 seconds.

- ☒ Every set that ranges from 12 to 15 repetitions should take approximately 48 to 60 seconds to complete—or an average of 54 seconds.

Certain exercises that require you to work each leg or arm independently—such as the lunge or the one-arm row—will take twice the amount of time to perform, but the amount of time you'll rest between sets will still be the same.

Take a rest. Resting between sets gives your muscles time to remove excess lactic acid—a chemical by-product of exercise responsible for that burning sensation in your muscles. However, the amount of time you should rest between sets depends on how much weight you're lifting. The heavier the weight—or resistance—you use, the more time your muscles need to recover.

Generally, after performing a set of 8 to 12 repetitions, the waiting time is no more than 30 to 60 seconds. (For 12 to 15 repetitions, rest 15 to 30 seconds; for 6 to 8 repetitions, rest 60 to 90 seconds.) However, in situations where you may have less—or even more—time to exercise, the amount of time you spend resting may vary slightly. For example, resting less than is required means you won't be able to lift as much weight during sets, but it may help you squeeze in more exercises during the limited time you have. Decreasing time between sets also trains your body more aerobically, helping to improve your cardiovascular health and burn fat. Resting more—up to 2 minutes—may make your workout longer, but it allows your muscles to recover more so they're stronger for the next set. Because this book contains 120 routines that utilize all of these principles, it's important to know your basics, but realize that you may be going off the menu for certain routines.

Once you know how long each set of an exercise should take you—as well as how long you should rest between sets—it's easy to figure out how many sets you can fit into whatever time you have to exercise. Take a look at how easily your workouts break down.

6 TO 8 REPETITIONS PER SET

For routines that use exercises that require 6 to 8 repetitions per set, the average time it should take you to complete 1 set is 28 seconds. That means . . .

. . . rest 30 seconds between each set and you should be able to do . . .

- ☒ 1 set in 58 seconds
- ☒ 10 sets in under 10 minutes
- ☒ 20 sets in under 20 minutes
- ☒ 30 sets in under 30 minutes
- ☒ 45 sets in under 45 minutes
- ☒ 60 sets in under 60 minutes

. . . rest 45 seconds between each set and you should be able to do . . .

- ☒ 1 set in 73 seconds
- ☒ 8 sets in under 10 minutes
- ☒ 16 sets in under 20 minutes
- ☒ 24 sets in under 30 minutes
- ☒ 36 sets in under 45 minutes
- ☒ 49 sets in under 60 minutes

. . . rest 60 seconds between each set and you should be able to do . . .

- ☒ 1 set in 88 seconds
- ☒ 6 sets in under 10 minutes
- ☒ 13 sets in under 20 minutes
- ☒ 20 sets in under 30 minutes
- ☒ 30 sets in under 45 minutes
- ☒ 40 sets in under 60 minutes

. . . rest 90 seconds between each set and you should be able to do . . .

- ☒ 1 set in 2 minutes
- ☒ 5 sets in under 10 minutes
- ☒ 10 sets in under 20 minutes
- ☒ 15 sets in under 30 minutes
- ☒ 23 sets in just over 45 minutes
- ☒ 30 sets in under 60 minutes

. . . rest 2 minutes between each set and you should be able to do . . .

- ☒ 1 set in 2 minutes, 28 seconds
- ☒ 4 sets in under 10 minutes
- ☒ 8 sets in under 20 minutes
- ☒ 12 sets in under 30 minutes
- ☒ 18 sets in under 45 minutes
- ☒ 24 sets in under 60 minutes

8 TO 12 REPETITIONS PER SET

For routines that use exercises that require 8 to 12 repetitions per set, the average time it should take you to complete 1 set is 40 seconds. That means . . .

. . . rest 15 seconds between each set and you should be able to do . . .

- ☒ 1 set in 55 seconds
- ☒ 10 sets in under 10 minutes
- ☒ 21 sets in under 20 minutes
- ☒ 32 sets in under 30 minutes
- ☒ 49 sets in under 45 minutes
- ☒ 65 sets in under 60 minutes

. . . rest 30 seconds between each set and you should be able to do . . .

- ☒ 1 set in 70 seconds
- ☒ 8 sets in under 10 minutes
- ☒ 17 sets in under 20 minutes
- ☒ 25 sets in under 30 minutes

☒ 38 sets in under 45 minutes

☒ 51 sets in under 60 minutes

...rest 45 seconds between each set and you should be able to do...

☒ 1 set in 85 seconds

☒ 6 sets in under 10 minutes

☒ 13 sets in under 20 minutes

☒ 20 sets in under 30 minutes

☒ 30 sets in under 45 minutes

☒ 40 sets in under 60 minutes

...rest 60 seconds between each set and you should be able to do...

☒ 1 set in 100 seconds

☒ 6 sets in under 10 minutes

☒ 12 sets in under 20 minutes

☒ 18 sets in under 30 minutes

☒ 27 sets in under 45 minutes

☒ 36 sets in under 60 minutes

...rest 90 seconds between each set and you should be able to do...

☒ 1 set in 2 minutes, 10 seconds

☒ 5 sets in just over 10 minutes

☒ 9 sets in under 20 minutes

☒ 13 sets in under 30 minutes

☒ 20 sets in under 45 minutes

☒ 27 sets in under 60 minutes

12 TO 15 REPETITIONS PER SET

For routines that use exercises that require 12 to 15 repetitions per set, the average time it should take you to complete 1 set is 54 seconds. That means...

...rest 15 seconds between each set and you should be able to do...

☒ 1 set in 69 seconds

☒ 8 sets in under 10 minutes

☒ 17 sets in under 20 minutes

☒ 25 sets in under 30 minutes

☒ 38 sets in under 45 minutes

☒ 51 sets in under 60 minutes

...rest 30 seconds between each set and you should be able to do...

☒ 1 set in 84 seconds

☒ 6 sets in under 10 minutes

☒ 13 sets in under 20 minutes

☒ 20 sets in under 30 minutes

☒ 30 sets in under 45 minutes

☒ 40 sets in under 60 minutes

...rest 45 seconds between each set and you should be able to do...

☒ 1 set in 99 seconds

☒ 6 sets in under 10 minutes

☒ 12 sets in under 20 minutes

☒ 18 sets in under 30 minutes

☒ 27 sets in under 45 minutes

☒ 36 sets in under 60 minutes

...rest 60 seconds between each set and you should be able to do...

☒ 1 set in 114 seconds

☒ five sets in under 10 minutes

☒ 10 sets in under 20 minutes

☒ 15 sets in under 30 minutes

☒ 23 sets in under 45 minutes

☒ 30 sets in under 60 minutes

ONCE YOU'RE DONE STRENGTH TRAINING . . .

Pay attention to your pain. Experiencing muscle soreness during or following a workout is normal. In fact, it means you're getting a good workout. Contracting a muscle past its threshold causes waste material and other acids to build up inside of it. Experiencing this burning sensation means your muscles are getting their money's worth.

If you feel a muscle begin to cramp, stop what you're doing and gently stretch the muscle until it unwinds itself. However, if you feel any sharp, continuous pain during exercise, or pain that persists after a few days, stop lifting and get yourself checked out by a doctor to be on the safe side.

Pay attention to your numbers. Keeping track of your exercise is just as important to your future as tracking your expenses. The fastest way to see results is by challenging the muscles with every workout. But you'll never accomplish this if you can't remember how hard you worked them the day before.

Write down every detail about each workout—how much weight you used, how many sets and repetitions you did, and so on—and refer back to it at the beginning of your next workout.

Pay attention to your plan. Muscles adapt to stress quickly, adjusting themselves within six to eight workouts to perform more efficiently. Eventually, your body learns to perform these moves using less energy and less stress, making the routine less effective for building muscle. Sticking with any specific routine for a long period of time also increases your odds of developing an overuse injury.

Keep your muscles guessing by changing your routine every 3 to 4 weeks, even if things are going smoothly. This doesn't have to mean an exercise overhaul. Just changing the weight or adding a new exercise mixes up a routine enough to feel

CHEAT SHEET

Timing is everything, especially when it comes to how much you spend on your muscles. Here's a quick checklist so you'll always know how to lift weights when minutes matter.

If you're strength training for muscular size and power . . .

☒ Lift the weight: 6 to 8 repetitions in each set.
☒ Rest: 60 to 90 seconds between sets.

If you're strength training for a combination of leanness, strength, and size . . .

☒ Lift the weight: 8 to 12 repetitions in each set.
☒ Rest: 30 to 60 seconds between sets.

If you're strength training for muscular endurance and a leaner look . . .

☒ Lift the weight: 12 to 15 repetitions in each set.
☒ Rest: 15 to 30 seconds between sets.

different to your body. With 120 workouts in this book, you'll have no trouble mixing things up so that the results keep on coming.

The Muscles You're Trying to Change

All muscles are not created equal.

Working out your chest, biceps, and back on a regular basis may be the fastest way to forge a body that looks built for anything. But if your goal is to have a body that truly *is* built for anything, you have to cover all your bases. As I mentioned earlier, if you neglect certain muscle groups in favor of more aesthetically pleasing ones, you can easily disrupt how efficiently your body divides work within itself. The result is a body that ends up overusing its weaker muscles while underutilizing its stronger muscles. Muscle fatigue, soreness, loss of stamina, and overuse injuries are just a handful of ways your body may "thank" you for this neglect. But the real crime comes from not letting your body develop to its full potential.

An exercise routine that focuses on every muscle group equally is crucial for getting your body to look—and perform—at its absolute best. If you're ready for a body like that, then let me introduce you to each and every muscle group personally.

In the Front (from head to toe!)

YOUR SHOULDERS

What you should know about them: Your shoulders are actually made up of three separate muscles, or *heads.* The anterior and medial heads (located on the front and sides of your shoulders, consecutively) begin on your collar bone. The posterior head (which makes up the back part of your shoulders) attaches on your *scapula,* or shoulder blade. All three heads wrap over and join by attaching to your *humerus,* or upper arm bone.

What your body expects them to do: Your shoulders basically are in charge of moving your arms away from your torso. Each head works differently from the others: Your anterior head lifts each arm up in front of your body; your medial head raises each arm out to your sides; your posterior head lifts each arm up and behind you.

Bonus: How building them makes you look even better! Combined with a well-developed back, a pair of stronger, broader shoulders can help widen your upper body, creating the illusion of a thinner waist. They also help out other muscles—especially your chest and back

and triceps—during different exercises that work those muscles. Training your shoulders can prevent them from tiring out too soon, so you can exhaust your chest and back muscles more thoroughly for more development.

YOUR CHEST

What you should know about it: The *pectoralis major* and *pectoralis minor* are the two major muscles that make up your chest. Your pectoralis major is a fan-shaped muscle that starts wide at the center of your body, stretches across each side of your chest, and thins out to connect to your upper arm bones. Beneath it lies your pectoralis minor, a thinner muscle that starts at your ribs and also connects to the upper arm.

> MUSCLES ADAPT TO STRESS QUICKLY, ADJUSTING THEMSELVES WITHIN SIX TO EIGHT WORKOUTS TO PERFORM MORE EFFICIENTLY. EVENTUALLY, YOUR BODY LEARNS TO PERFORM THESE MOVES USING LESS ENERGY AND LESS STRESS, MAKING THE ROUTINE LESS EFFECTIVE FOR BUILDING MUSCLE.

What your body expects it to do: Your chest muscles have the job of moving your arms inward and across your body at various angles.

YOUR BICEPS

What you should know about them: Your biceps are actually two separate muscles that both attach at the shoulder socket and insert onto your *radius*—one of the two bones within your forearms. Between your biceps and your upper arm bone is the *brachialis,* a thin muscle that attaches to the *ulna*—the other bone within your forearms.

What your body expects them to do:
Your biceps' main duty is to bend your elbows—or, basically, to move your lower arms toward your shoulders. They also rotate your lower arms from side to side, which turns your palms from an up to a down position and vice versa.

YOUR FOREARMS

What you should know about them:
There are two sets of muscles within your forearms. The *flexors,* located on the palm side of your forearms, start at the end of your humerus bone and end at your hands. The extensors, found along the other side of your forearms, also start at the humerus bone and end at your hands.

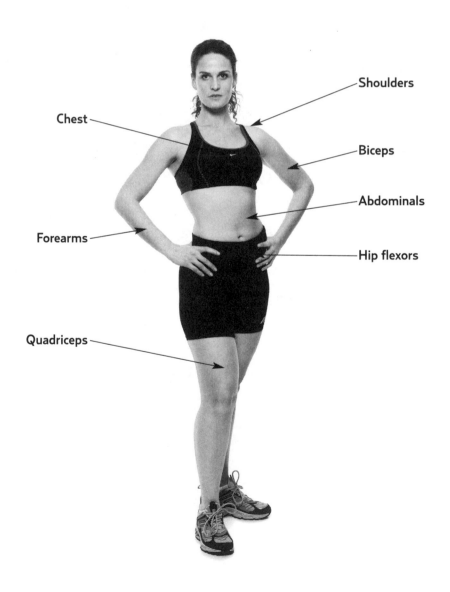

Chest

Shoulders

Biceps

Abdominals

Forearms

Hip flexors

Quadriceps

What your body expects them to do:
Your flexors pull your wrists forward—or, in other words, draw your hand down—while your extensors pull your wrists back.

Bonus: How building them makes you look even better! No one thinks twice about spending much effort on these tiny muscles, which still manage to get a good workout during many exercises that require a strong grip. But if you have the time, focusing on these muscles can help you get more from most exercises that work your back and biceps muscles. That's because they are equally important in providing a strong grip—critical for all the pulling and curling motions that most back and biceps exercises require.

YOUR ABDOMINALS

What you should know about them:
Your abdominals are actually composed of four separate muscle groups—the *rectus abdominis,* the *external and internal obliques,* and the *transverse abdominis.* Your rectus abdominis—the muscle responsible for that "six-pack" look—runs from your breastbone to your pubic bone. Your internal and external obliques are paired along each side of your waist and lie diagonally across your midsection. Your transverse abdominis muscle hides deep beneath your external and internal obliques.

What your body expects them to do: The primary job of your rectus abdominis is to pull your torso toward your hips. Your obliques work together to rotate your torso from side to side, as well as to bend your torso in toward your hips. Finally, your transverse abdominis keeps your entire abdominal wall drawn inward, which protects your internal organs while it helps support your spine.

YOUR HIP FLEXORS

What you should know about them: Located in the front of your thighs, your hip flexors are actually two muscle groups: the *iliacus* and the

psoas major (collectively referred to as the *iliopsoas muscle*). The iliacus starts at your pelvis and attaches to your thighbone, while the psoas major starts on your lumbar vertebrae and also connects to your thighbone.

What your body expects them to do:
The hip flexors' main job is to draw your thighs toward your midsection.

Bonus: How building them makes you look even better! Even though they're not really a muscle group you can see, developing them can help you get more from other popular exercises that work other muscle groups. The stronger and looser you can make your hip flexors, the easier it is for them to extend your leg out as far as possible. The result is a wider stride that can increase your speed significantly when running. Working these tiny stabilizers also keeps your pelvis in perfect alignment with your spine while doing certain abdominal exercises.

YOUR QUADRICEPS

What you should know about them: Your quadriceps—the muscles that rest along the front of your thighs—divide into four separate groups: the *vastus intermedius,* the *rectus femoris,* the *vastus lateralis,* and the *vastus medialis.* They attach at the top of your thighbone, run down your thigh toward your knee, and end at the top of your shinbone.

What your body expects them to do:
Your quadriceps' main role is to straighten your legs, but they also come into play to support the inner and outer sides of your knee joints.

Bonus: How building them makes you look even better! Paying enough attention to these stabilizing muscles can lower your risk of developing knee pain or injury. If fat loss is your goal, that means more time to cycle, run, or walk pain-free.

In the Back (from head to toe!)

YOUR TRAPEZIUS

What you should know about it: This flat, triangular-shaped muscle starts at the base of your skull and inserts itself at the back of your collarbone and shoulder blades, adding shape to the upper part of your neck and shoulders.

What your body expects it to do: This muscle helps draw your shoulder blades together as well as pull them down. It's also responsible for your ability to shrug your arms upward.

YOUR RHOMBOIDS

What you should know about them: Hidden directly beneath your trapezius, your rhomboids lie in the middle of your upper back—right between your shoulder blades.

What your body expects them to do: Your rhomboids assist your trapezius in pulling your shoulder blades toward each other.

YOUR LATISSIMUS DORSI

What you should know about them: Your latissimus dorsi are a set of fan-shaped mus-

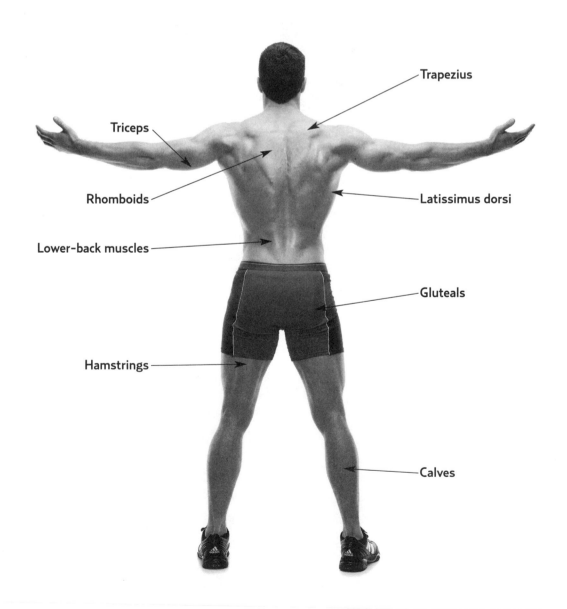

Triceps

Trapezius

Rhomboids

Latissimus dorsi

Lower-back muscles

Gluteals

Hamstrings

Calves

BUILDING YOUR LATISSIMUS DORSI MUSCLES CAN GIVE YOUR BACK A WIDER, FLARED APPEARANCE THAT TAPERS DOWN TO YOUR WAIST, CREATING A V-SHAPE SYMMETRY THAT MAKES YOUR BODY LOOK SMALLER AT ITS CENTER.

cles found along the sides of your body. They start low on your spine, spread across the width of your back, and taper off at your upper arm bone (where it meets your shoulders).

What your body expects them to do: The main job required of your latissimus dorsi—or "lats"—is to pull your arms down from an upward position above your shoulders. When your arms are extended in front of your torso, they also are responsible for pulling your arms toward your torso.

Bonus: How building them makes you look even better! Your lats are the largest muscles of your back, so shaping up this large body of real estate can make a huge difference in how you look from behind. Building these muscles can give your back a wider, flared appearance that tapers down to your waist, creating a V-shape symmetry that makes your body look smaller at its center.

YOUR LOWER-BACK MUSCLES

What you should know about them: Beginning at the back of your skull and ending at your pelvis, your *erector spinae*—or spinal erectors—are two columns of muscle, one on each side of your spine.

What your body expects them to do: The job of your erector spinae muscles is to straighten out your spine after you bend forward, and also to keep it in an upright position so that you maintain proper posture all day long. These muscles are also responsible for letting you bend your torso backward into an arched position.

Bonus: How building them makes you look even better! Your erector spinae muscles continuously support your spine to improve your posture whenever you walk, run, or do any exercise that requires a straight back. Making them stronger also lets them disguise your sagging belly. Standing straight and holding in your stomach takes strong, resilient muscles along the spine and throughout the lower back. The stronger these muscles are, the easier it is for them to keep your back straight throughout the day.

YOUR TRICEPS

What you should know about them: Your triceps are made up of three separate muscles—the lateral head, the medial head, and the long head. The lateral and medial heads both start at your upper arm bone, while the long head starts at your shoulder blades. All three come together and attach to a tendon that connects to your elbow bone, or *ulna*.

What your body expects them to do: Your triceps' job is to straighten your arms by extending your elbows. They also assist with other, secondary tasks, from stabilizing your shoulder joints during certain movements to helping your upper back muscles whenever you pull your arms down and behind your body.

Bonus: How building them makes you look even better: Most people looking to develop their arms spend all their efforts on their biceps. However, your triceps make up more than 60 percent of the muscles in your upper arm, which means they actually deserve more of your attention. Developing your triceps to their full potential can also give you more strength during exercises where they assist other muscles, including many exercises that work your chest and shoulder muscles.

YOUR GLUTEALS

What you should know about them: The muscles that make up your butt are divided into three groups: the *gluteus maximus, medius,* and *minimus.* Your gluteus maximus—one of the largest and strongest muscles—starts at your pelvic bone and connects to the back of your thighbone. Your medius and minimus also start at your pelvic bone but end along the sides of your thighbone.

What your body expects them to do: Your gluteus maximus assists your hamstrings to draw your leg straight back behind you, while your gluteus medius and minimus work together to raise your leg out to the side.

YOUR HAMSTRINGS

What you should know about them: Your hamstrings make up the entire musculature of the back of your thighs. Made up of three separate muscles, they all attach at your pelvic bone, stretch down each thigh, and insert either on your shinbone or the head of your fibula—a tiny bone on your lower leg.

What your body expects them to do: Your hamstrings' two main tasks are to flex, or bend, your knees and to extend your hips (the movement you make when you kick your leg back behind you).

YOUR CALVES

What you should know about them: You have two sets of muscles below your knees: the *gastrocnemius* and the *soleus* muscles. The gastrocnemius rides higher along the back of your lower legs and is the "rounded" muscle you see along the outer sides of your calves. Your soleus is flatter and rests below the gastrocnemius.

What your body expects them to do: Both your gastrocnemius and soleus muscles' main task is to point your toes down, plus assist in flexing your knees.

Bonus: How building them makes you look even better! Most people tend to forget these muscles, but your lower legs—along with your arms—are typically one of the most exposed muscle groups you have. Paying them the attention they deserve can keep your legs from looking too thin the next time you're wearing shorts.

Many of the exercises that target the quadriceps also involve your calves. Strengthening them can keep them from burning out too soon, so you can train your quadriceps longer for faster results.

The Tools You Need for Doing the Job

With thousands of exercise machines, gadgets, and accessories out there promising to rebuild your body with amazing results, you would think that you're in for the largest chapter of the book, right?

Wrong.

You can't write a book that gives its readers complete freedom to change their workouts on a dime, then expect them to have every piece of exercise equipment imaginable at their disposal. Granted, if you have access to a gym or a club, you have access to everything you'll need for getting the most from this book. If you don't, then don't worry. All you need for doing nearly every single workout in this book is yourself, an exercise bench, and an adjustable pair of dumbbells.

Still, if you're in the mood to invest more in your muscles, it pays to know how to pick your exercise equipment in the right order. You see, setting up a home gym is like starting a new relationship. Those high-priced, multigadgeted infomercial machines you see at 2:30 in the morning may look tempting, but what doesn't look good when you're sleep-deprived at 2:30 in the morning? Most of them will break your heart (not to mention your bank account) and never live up to your expectations. Rush into things too quickly and you risk ending up confused, bitter, and broke.

Before you spend your hard-earned money, the key is taking the time to slowly get to know exercise just as you would a person. What to buy—and how much to spend—all depends on what stage you're in with exercise at the time.

STEP 1: DETERMINE HOW MUCH YOU CAN AFFORD TO LOSE

Purchasing fitness equipment based on hyped promises or 10 easy payment plans can lead to a room filled with machines that give you less results for your dollar. To be on the safe side, you want to be sure that if you lose your motivation to exercise down the road, you don't end up losing your shirt like many exercise-equipment purchasers do.

Before you start using this book to succeed, I want you to imagine that you're about to fail instead. Then, look at your bank account with a careful eye. Come up with a set price of how much money you can afford to lose, and let that be the starting point of how much you can afford to spend. Once you stay on track for at least 3 months, you can easily spend more.

STEP 2: BUY EQUIPMENT IN THE RIGHT ORDER

Creating a home gym that can handle the exercise prescriptions in this book doesn't mean having to spend a lot of money. But it does require that you have enough of the right essentials to deliver a total-body workout.

You want to start slow and buy in the right order, according to your level of commitment. Purchasing a set of adjustable free weights and an exercise bench lets you do hundreds of exercises, which is wiser than buying some high-tech exercise machine that may look nicer in your den but lets you do only a handful of challenging moves. That also goes for big, expensive cardiovascular machines, such as treadmills and elliptical machines. Let a pricey treadmill or elliptical trainer be the reward for meeting your goals, not the solution for working toward your goals.

Now that you know your budget, here's how to buy your equipment in the right order.

The Beginner (Zero to 6 months)

Forget about wining and dining at this stage. The simplest things impress your body during the early stages of exercise. Every time feels like the first time, and it doesn't take much effort to turn exercise on and see instant results.

Here's all you'll need to invest in.

One pair of adjustable dumbbells: The building-block exercises to an impressive physique—chest presses, chest flies, one-arm rows, shoulder presses, biceps curls, triceps extensions, lunges, and squats—can all be done using nothing more than this. Warning: Avoid time-consuming weight collars that require tools or unscrewing to remove them, and opt for a pair of spring-release or Quicklee collars instead (both types slide on, lock in place, and slide off with just a squeeze). Average cost: $35 to $50 for the dumbbells, $5 to $15 for the collars.

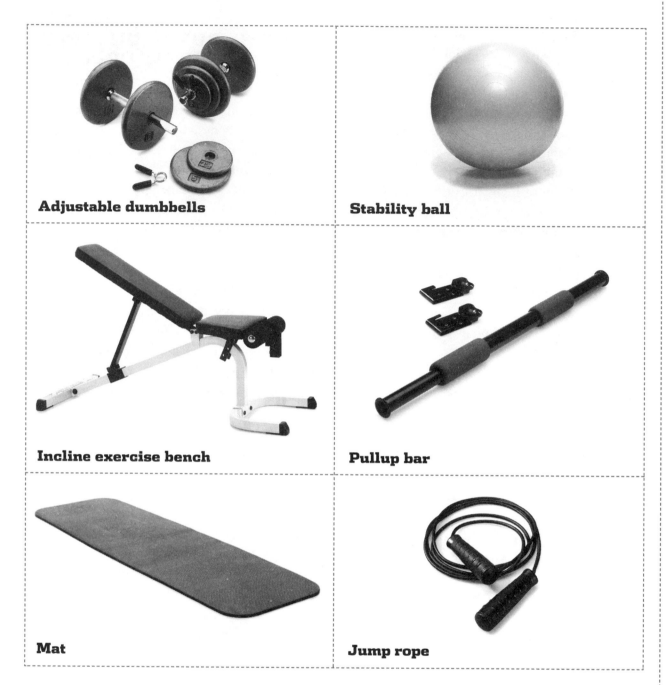

Adjustable dumbbells

Stability ball

Incline exercise bench

Pullup bar

Mat

Jump rope

An exercise bench that inclines: Without one, it's nearly impossible to work your chest. Average cost: $60 to $100.

A mat: Crunches are painful enough without grinding your spine on bad shag carpeting. Average cost: $10 to $20.

A stability ball: Offers dozens of exercises for toning, strengthening, and stretching. Average cost: $20 to $40.

A pullup bar: Most people make the mistake of bypassing pullups for a lat-pulldown station instead, but pullups are the fastest way to a strong, broad back. Average cost: $15 to $30.

A jump rope: It takes up less space than an empty beer bottle and it burns up to 800 calories an hour. That's more than you can expect to burn on a treadmill, at 1/100 the price. Average cost: $5 to $20.

TOTAL COMMITMENT: $150 to $275.

The Intermediate
(6 months to 3 years)

Around this time, the magic can wear off for your muscles. The same moves that used to leave your muscles impressed enough to grow barely have them sore the next morning. You need something to spice things up, fast. Keep all your beginner equipment, but realize that it's time to add the following:

An Olympic barbell set: The advantage of lifting with a bar is that you can use heavier weight than you can with dumbbells. More weight equals bigger muscles. Instead of buying a bar and weight plates separately, look for a package deal. Most manufacturers sell 300-pound sets that come with all the trimmings—a bar, a range of weight plates, and a pair of collars. Again, ask for collars that slide on and off to save time. Average cost: $100 to $200.

An exercise bench that inclines and declines (with optional leg curl/extension attachment): The leg attachment will give you more variety in your leg routine besides squats and lunges, and having more range when it comes to the angle of the bench can help you target certain muscle groups more thoroughly. If you really want to make an investment, an Olympic-style bench is a better bet. These benches tend to be sturdier than an average bench, plus most feature a rack system wide enough to accommodate a 6-foot-long Olympic bar—perfect when doing barbell presses and other power exercises. Average cost: $200 to $500.

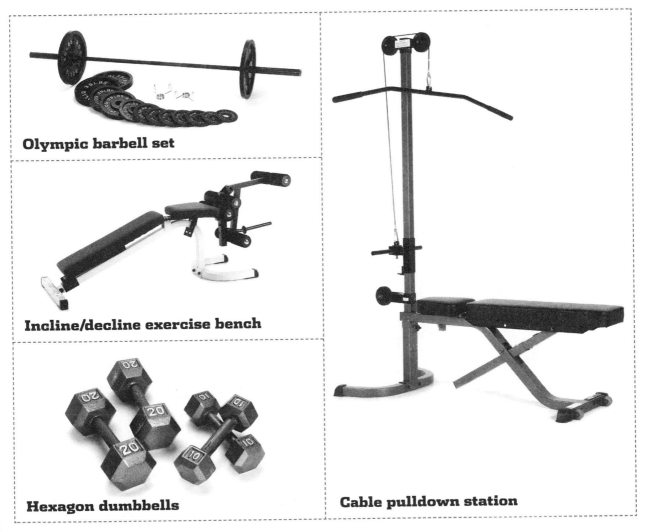

Olympic barbell set

Incline/decline exercise bench

Hexagon dumbbells

Cable pulldown station

One or two pairs of hexagon dumbbells: By now, you've discovered which weight settings you use most frequently, so invest in a pair of fixed-weight dumbbells. That way, you can grab and go instead of having to whip out your abacus and a new stack of plates every time you need to adjust the weight. Average cost: $50.

A cable pulldown station: A single pulley tower can be affixed where your leg attachment attaches to your bench. Although this tool is primarily for working your back, with a little creativity, you can also build your triceps, biceps, and shoulders. Average cost: $50 to 80.

TOTAL COMMITMENT: $400 to more than $800.

The Advanced
(3 years and beyond)

By now, you know everything there is to know about exercise, and familiarity has certainly bred contempt. It has also bred stalled progress. Inevitably, you have to lay down some money to show that you're ready for a lifetime commitment.

Variety is now more important than ever, and equipping yourself with a few new toys will allow you to experiment more than ever before. Besides, now's the time to spend money with confidence. Three years is a long time. You've been together too long to let exercise slip out of your life. So take a deep breath, take a deeper dig into your wallet, and spend some money on your future.

You should have everything the beginner and intermediate has, with the following additions:

An assortment of fixed-weight dumbbells: Your adjustable ones are history now, since it's harder to combine exercises or experiment with shorter rests between sets if you're constantly reloading weights. Pass these iron torches on to your little brother and buy pairs of dumbbells from 5 pounds up to the highest

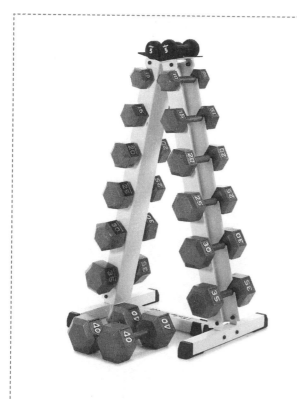

Fixed-weight dumbbells

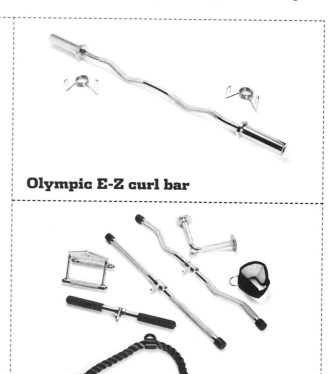

Olympic E-Z curl bar

Cable attachments

YOU HAVE THE TIME, BUT DO YOU HAVE THE ROOM?

Most experts agree that having a separate room to exercise in is the best way to stay motivated. The catch-22 is that people typically use whatever unusable space they have in their homes, which typically means the least attractive room in the house. Instead of picking whatever room in the house is vacant, ask yourself these five questions first. If you can say yes to all five, then you've found the room that's perfect for you.

1. Is there enough space to play in? You need to make sure you have enough space for what you'll be filling the room with but also for any new equipment you may invest in later on. Don't forget to figure out the floor-to-ceiling space if you're considering a fitness machine down the line (some have attachments that can reach 6 to 7 feet off the ground).

The following guidelines from the American Council on Exercise can help you figure out how much space you'll need:

☒ Treadmill: 30 square feet

☒ Stationary bike: 10 square feet

☒ Free weights: 20 to 50 square feet

☒ Exercise mat: 12 square feet

☒ Single-station gym: 35 square feet

☒ Stairclimber: 10 to 20 square feet

☒ Multistation gym: 50 to 200 square feet

2. Is there enough light? Pick a room with as much natural light as possible. Studies have shown that darkness places your body in a relaxed mood that makes it harder to exercise.

3. Are there enough windows? Raising your heart rate from exercise forces your body to use more oxygen. That's why a well-ventilated area is best for exercise. If you have no choice but to use a windowless area, make sure there's enough room to invest in a few strong fans to keep the air flowing freely.

4. Are there enough electrical outlets? You'll need access to electricity for fans, cardiovascular machines, entertainment equipment, and so on.

5. Is the floor sturdy enough? The room should have a floor that can support the weight of a treadmill, weight station, or any other heavy machine you may want to add. If the room is above another room, invest in some heavy, commercial-grade carpeting and rubber pads to keep moisture from soaking into the floor and to muffle the noise.

weight you're currently using, building in 5-pound increments. Average cost: $350 to $450, for dumbbells from 5 to 50 pounds.

One Olympic E-Z curl bar: Bent in the center, this bar angles your wrists as you curl, press (during triceps extensions), or pull (during upright rows) to alleviate excess strain and avoid repetitive-use injuries common from years of working out. Average cost: $60 to $100.

A variety of cable attachments: From dual-end ropes and close-grip bars to single arm handles and V-shaped pulldown bars, these help work your muscles from different angles for a more thorough workout. Average cost: $20 to $30 each.

Cardio machine: Blowing a few paychecks on a machine is perfectly legitimate now, but put some thought into what to buy. If you have bad knees, go with a high-end cycle. If you have no backside, go with a stairclimber. If you have the space, go with a treadmill. Average cost: From as little as $100 to as high as $5,000, depending on what you buy.

TOTAL COMMITMENT: More than $500 to as high as $5,500.

Spend More Time . . . Talking to Yourself!

Don't even have the time—or maybe the patience—to keep track of your pulse? That's okay, because you can use your voice to figure out whether you're getting a good workout instead. As you exercise, try carrying on a conversation, even if it's with yourself. If you can do that with no problem, odds are you're not challenging your cardiovascular system enough to reap the kind of aerobic benefits you're looking for. Once you reach a point where it becomes difficult to hold a conversation and exercise at the same time, then you'll be pushing yourself at an intensity that's within your aerobic threshold.

The Results You're Looking to See

It may be hard for you to predict what your schedule will look like from week to week, but it's even more difficult for me to venture a guess at what type of physique you're hoping to build. That's why this book is going to give you a choice between four of them.

You heard me.

Four physiques.

Are you looking to lose weight and slim down?

Are you hoping to chisel a body of solid, lean muscle?

Are you in it purely to get your muscles as strong and as powerful as possible?

Or would you like a more versatile physique that's a mixture of all three?

Guess what? We have you covered no matter what.

Chapters 5 through 10 of this book will break down exactly what you should do, depending on how many days of the week you have to exercise: 1, 2, 3, 4, 5, or 6 days. (If you have 7 days, hold on—we'll get to you in chapter 11.) In each of those chapters, you'll find five subsections with different types of workouts to use, depending on the amount of time you have (10, 20, 30, 45, or 60 minutes). That's a total of 30 subsections of workouts available whenever you need them.

But, to make sure you can meet your goals, I've gone a step further. Each of the 30 subsections offers four different workouts to choose from—one for building lean muscle, one for weight loss, one for muscle power, and one that gives you the best of all three. That's a total of 120 time-effective workouts, each specifically created to match your current goals!

Here's how—and why—it works.

1. Were you the one looking to lose weight and slim down? Then whenever you decide how many days and minutes you can spare—in that specific section—you should choose:

Your Instant Lean-Body Plan!

Weight loss is the number one reason men and women alike bother to exercise, which is why this workout is the top choice to turn to among all the routines in this book. It's also one of the most misunderstood methods of exercise—but don't worry, it's easy if you know the basics.

The smartest exercises for burning calories employ less resistance, targeting slow-twitch fibers within your muscles that are capable of performing continuously for extended periods of time. Raising the amount of repetitions in each set to 12 to 15, plus choosing more body part–specific exercises to isolate your muscles, is a trick that even most bodybuilders use to decrease their body fat and tone/harden up their muscles.

Some workouts may claim to add definition to your muscles, but muscular definition is really a combination of building lean muscle tissue and reducing the amount of body fat and water that are covering your muscles up. Sticking to a program that uses more repetitions increases your body's caloric needs, which can help in lowering body fat.

Using a routine that limits how much rest your muscles get in between sets can also help burn fat by making your weight-lifting program more aerobic. Not giving your muscles an opportunity to rest between sets—or limiting the rest time to 15 to 30 seconds—strings exercises into a fast-moving workout that keeps your heart rate at a constant, elevated pace, similar to cardiovascular exercise. You'll notice that all 30 "instant lean-body plans" in this book are built upon a combination of all these principles.

Finally, if fat loss is truly your main goal, then get ready to expect your fair share of cardiovascular exercise to help burn calories. In fact, if you have minimal time or days to spare, you may find

RAISING THE AMOUNT OF REPETITIONS IN EACH SET TO 12 TO 15, PLUS CHOOSING MORE BODY PART–SPECIFIC EXERCISES TO ISOLATE YOUR MUSCLES, IS A TRICK THAT EVEN MOST BODY-BUILDERS USE TO DECREASE THEIR BODY FAT AND TONE/HARDEN UP THEIR MUSCLES.

that cardiovascular exercise is the *only* program prescribed for you that day. That's because nothing burns calories—and fat—more effectively than cardiovascular exercise. So don't be surprised if a routine requires you to burn excess calories and body fat over building muscle.

Starting on page 37, I'll tell you everything you need to know about cardiovascular, or *aerobic*, exercise. This section was written specifically with you in mind, and it relates to every program you'll be using, so read it carefully. If you can master the

rules revealed within it, you'll always work your heart at a pace that can help your body burn more calories in the shortest period of time.

2. Were you the one hoping to chisel a body of solid, lean muscle? Then whenever you decide how many days and minutes you can spare—in that specific section—you should choose:

Your Instant Muscle Plan!

If your goal is to improve the overall shape and size of your muscles toward a well-built body, then you're in luck. Achieving those goals is easy when you train your muscles in the correct way so they respond the way you want them to.

The most effective method uses exercises that isolate each muscle group. The less involvement other muscles have in each exercise, the faster the targeted muscles can respond. Always maintaining between 8 and 12 repetitions per set helps target the fast-twitch fibers within your muscles, fibers that are quicker to grow, so you can add shape to your frame much faster. Keeping your rest time to 30 to 90 seconds between sets is the ideal range to allow muscles just enough time to recover.

All 30 "instant muscle plans" in this book are designed with all these specifications in place, offering you the total peace of mind that each and every workout you turn to will give your body the muscle-shaping results it expects.

3. Was your goal purely to get your muscles as strong and as powerful as possible? Then whenever you decide how many days and minutes you can spare—in that specific section—you should choose:

Your Instant Power Plan!

Building powerful muscles that are less about size and more about strength means choosing exercises that give you the most bang for your buck. You need a routine of compound exercises that work several muscle groups at once, as opposed to exercises that isolate muscle groups individually. That's why a program designed for muscle mass is typically built around compound exercises—such as deadlifts, squats, and bench presses. These types of moves let you work with heavier amounts of weight, which helps to build muscle strength.

Training for power also means using free-weight exercises as opposed to exercise machines.

Why? Because unlike machine exercises, which tend to support your body or position it in a way that prevents other muscle groups from joining in, exercises using dumbbells and barbells recruit more muscle groups to help stabilize the body. Once again, all that extra help lets you handle heavier weight loads.

Handling larger amounts of weight also means your muscles may need extra time to recover between sets, which is why keeping your rest periods around 60 to 90 seconds—or even as long as several minutes—is critical for exercisers who are training for maximum strength.

RUN THE NUMBERS BEFORE YOU BOTHER SWEATING

Think all these numbers are too much to memorize? Now, you don't have to. Put the calculator down and use this handy chart instead. Just find your age, decide on what goal you are looking to accomplish, and keep your pulse between the numbers in that section.

Many experts agree that women have a higher maximum heart rate than men, but that doesn't mean women can't use this chart, too. If you're female, just add 6 to each of these numbers on this chart—except your age, of course!—and you'll also be able to get everything from your aerobic exercise, every time.

Your Age	Your MHR (beats per minute)	Stay Healthy (50–60% of MHR) (low intensity)	Burn More Fat (60–70% of MHR) (medium intensity)	Build More Endurance (70–80% of MHR) (high intensity)
20	200	100–120	120–140	140–160
25	195	97–117	117–137	137–156
30	190	95–114	114–133	133–152
35	185	92–111	111–129	129–148
40	180	90–108	108–126	126–144
45	175	87–105	105–122	122–140
50	170	85–102	102–119	119–136
55	165	82–99	99–115	115–132
60	160	80–96	96–112	112–128
65	155	77–93	93–108	108–124
70	150	75–90	90–105	105–120
75	145	72–87	87–101	101–116

TIME TWEAKS!

Spend Less Time . . . Counting Up Your Beats!

No one's expecting you to actually add up how many times your heart beats in 1 minute. Instead, take a shortcut: Place the tips of your middle finger and index finger—the finger that you point with—on the palm side of your other wrist, right below the base of the thumb. You can also take your pulse at your carotid artery, located right along either side of your neck.

Press gently, wait for a pulse, then start counting how many times your heart beats for 6 seconds. Multiply that number by 10 and you'll have the number you need for checking your level of intensity. If you are not within the zone you should be, adjust the intensity by speeding up or slowing down, raising or lowering the incline, and so on, and check again. Once you finally have your pulse in the zone where it should be, maintain those settings and check your pulse every few minutes to make sure your body stays there.

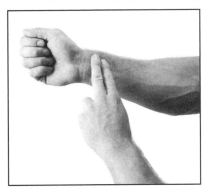 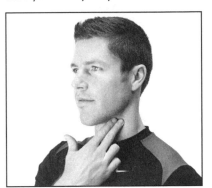

All 30 "instant power plans" in this book utilize all of these strength-building techniques, giving you everything you need for building muscles that are just as strong as they look.

Just don't be surprised if they end up even stronger!

4. Are you looking for a more versatile physique that's a mixture of all three—weight loss, muscle definition, and strength? Then whenever you decide how many days and minutes you can spare—in that specific section—you should choose:

Your Instant Complete-Body Plan!

Not every exerciser goes into his workout with a specific goal in mind. For some of us, the weight room is simply a means to a end. And for you, that end may just be getting all you can from your body, without having your brain get bored and quit on you in the process.

That's where these routines can become your escape from conventional exercise. All 30 "instant complete-body plans" in this book challenge you by using bits and pieces from the other three types of routines, so your body gets the best of all worlds. You'll also end up using the most-varied types of exercises in your routines, challenging your muscles from every angle for a physique that's always functional, no matter what sport, activity, or situation you find yourself looking to master.

Because you'll be performing certain programs from the "lean-body" routines, you'll need to know the fundamentals of cardiovascular exercise. Starting on page 37, I'll teach you all the rules you'll need for monitoring your heart to keep you burning more calories in the shortest period of time.

There's only one rule I'd like to stress: If you're just beginning to exercise, before trying the routines of the "complete-body plan," it's best to be familiar with the other three plans first. If you've been working out for at least 4 to 6 months, you should be ready to handle all the exciting variations these routines have to offer you.

TIME TWEAKS!

Spend Less Time . . . Wondering How You Should Sweat!

Even though most people associate running, cycling, and jumping rope with cardiovascular exercise, any activity—done at an elevated enough pace that challenges your heart and increases your body's need for oxygen—can classify as aerobic exercise.

If you're able to raise your heart rate and keep it in the zone recommended in the routine (50 to 60 percent of your MHR for low intensity; 60 to 70 percent of your MHR for medium intensity; 70 to 80 percent of your MHR for high intensity), then it doesn't matter to me—or your muscles—whether you're exercising in a gym or aerobic class, running on a track at the nearby high school, playing your favorite sport, or frantically yanking weeds from your garden.

However, there are still a few tried-and-true cardiovascular machines and activities you may want to rely on to get the job done. Knowing how to tweak these aerobic staples can be helpful the next time you need to increase the intensity to match the routines in this book.

Following are the basics on making five different kinds of cardiovascular exercise more intense—or even less intense—when necessary.

Running

Increase the intensity by . . . picking up the pace; running at a higher angle; running on sand, soft grass, or any stable, softer surface.

Lower the intensity by . . . lowering your speed; running on a flat surface; running for 10 seconds, then resting for 10 seconds (you can tailor the amount of rest between to lower it even further).

Avoid . . . relying on running downhill to lessen the intensity—exercising often at a grade steeper than 3 or 4 percent can aggravate your knees.

Walking

Increase the intensity by . . . moving at a brisker pace; walking at a higher angle; wearing a backpack with a light weight inside it.

Lower the intensity by . . . slowing down to a comfortable pace; walking on a level surface.

Avoid . . . adding hand weights or ankle weights. Doing so can affect your stride and put more stress on your knees and other joints.

Cycling

Increase the intensity by . . . pedaling faster; increasing your resistance (or grade); making sure you pull your feet up—instead of simply pushing them down—as you pedal.

Lower the intensity by . . . lowering your speed; cycling at a lower level of resistance (or grade); pedaling with one leg at a time.

Avoid . . . using too much resistance, which can bring on knee problems if your muscles aren't strong enough.

Jumping Rope

Increase the intensity by . . . jumping faster; rotating your arms farther from your body as you jump.

Lower the intensity by . . . jumping once or twice, resting for 2 to 3 seconds, then repeating.

Avoid . . . jumping higher—this just puts added stress on your knees.

Swimming

Increase the intensity by . . . swimming faster; choosing strokes that use both your arms and legs simultaneously.

Lower the intensity by . . . swimming at a slower pace; gliding through the water for a few seconds between strokes; turning your hands so that they cut through the water instead of catching water in your palms.

Avoid . . . training at a high intensity without proper supervision, especially outdoors. Swimming the length of the shoreline is always smarter than swimming forward into the water and back.

The One Muscle That Matters above Them All!

If you're the type who knows you'll be sticking to the "lean-body" and "complete-body" plans, you need to read this section before we start the program. Why? Because many of your routines will require you to perform some type of cardiovascular exercise in order to help burn fat and/or lose weight. If that sounds like what you'll be going after, you need to understand a few things about cardiovascular exercise before you try any of the routines.

And even if that's *not* your goal, you might still want to add a little cardio—or more than you're doing now—into your routines.

YOU'LL STAY AS YOUNG AS YOU FEEL

After you turn the big 3-o, your metabolism—the rate at which your body burns calories to function during the day—starts to slow down, causing you to store more excess calories as body fat. Most people put on about a pound of fat every year after they turn 30.

That's why it's so important to counteract that effect with some sort of cardiovascular, or aerobic, exercise. What qualifies as cardio or aerobic exercise? Any activity that elevates your heart rate and trains your lungs to become more efficient at delivering oxygen throughout your body.

But the benefits of cardio go beyond just burning a few extra calories. Cardio can keep you living longer, so you have more time to enjoy that new body you're going to spend so much time building up.

YOU'LL GIVE YOUR HEART A BREAK

Most people forget that the heart is a muscle that's easily improved through exercise. In fact, working your heart can make the rest of your muscles function even better during the routines you'll be using in this book. Strengthening your heart enables it to pump even more oxygen-rich blood throughout your body with less effort. If you're using the "lean-body" or "complete-body" plans, that extra boost is just what your muscles need to stick it out through many of those challenging routines.

Regular cardiovascular exercise has also been

TIME TWEAKS!

Spend More Time . . . Fine-Tuning Your Routines!

Stop throwing surprises at your muscles on a regular basis and they'll gladly stay the same, instead of developing into what you need them to be. Now, thanks to this book, you have 120 workouts to mix things up when you need to, but that doesn't mean you can't tweak

them even further. Try these two tactics with any of the 120 routines and you'll always get more from them—no matter which one you choose.

Try sitting once in a while. Some standing exercises, such as dumbbell presses and curls, can be more effectively performed in a seated position. This prevents you from cheating with your back muscles and isolates the muscles you want to work. (Rule of thumb when sitting: Lower the

weight by about 20 percent of what you normally use.) Don't have a seat to sit on? Then kneel instead—just be sure to keep your back straight and always in line with your thighs.

Try stopping once in a while. As you exercise, pause in the middle of lowering or raising the weight, hold for a second, then finish the movement. Doing this at any time helps exhaust your muscles even faster, and it also develops more balance and coordination.

shown to raise the amount of good cholesterol (HDL) and lower the levels of bad cholesterol (LDL) in your body—two health benefits that research has proven can lower your risk of heart disease. From a health standpoint, your odds of dealing with diabetes, hypertension, and many different forms of cancer down the road can all be lowered by just paying your heart the same attention as your other muscles.

YOU DON'T NEED TO BE AN EXPERT TO START SWEATING

Whether you opt to do any form of aerobic exercise is entirely dependent on your goals, but if you decide to add some cardio to your workouts, there are certain measurements already in place. Research has shown that the ideal for aerobic conditioning is to do some sort of cardiovascular exercise at a medium-intensity level at least 3 days a week, for 20 minutes a day. That doesn't mean you can't do less or more than that, depending on your schedule, but did you know that there's a way that you can tweak your aerobic exercise to make sure it matches your specific exercise goals?

If you're thinking of using the "instant muscle" or "instant power" plans, then you're probably so concerned with packing on muscle that you wouldn't want to risk burning off too many excess calories. Still, there is a way to do some type of cardiovascular exercise that's strictly for your health.

If you're going to start with the "instant leanbody" plan, you need to modify your cardiovascular workouts so that you always burn calories from the stored fat you're desperately trying to get rid of.

If you're opting to try the "instant complete-body" plan, you may be looking for a body that's not only lean but that also functions as well as it looks. Improving your endurance and stamina is the focus, and it's easily doable if you know how.

THE ONLY NUMBER YOU NEED TO KNOW

First, you need to do a little math for me. Write down 220 on a sheet of paper, then subtract your age from that number. (For example, if you're 30, then the number you should have come up with is 190.) This is the *only number you need to know* in order to use cardio exercise to your advantage. That number is your *maximum heart rate*—or MHR—the maximum number of beats per minute that your heart should be beating. (The most accurate version of your MHR is something that only an exercise stress test can determine, but this short, sweet rule-of-thumb is the standard most trainers use.)

Exercising hard enough to elevate your heart rate to a certain percentage of your MHR is all cardiovascular exercise really is. Your heart is conditioned and your body burns calories no matter where your heart rate falls as you exercise. But how high you decide to raise—and maintain—your pulse is what decides the results you get for all your efforts.

Fifty to 60 percent of your MHR: Keeping your pulse at this level is considered "low-intensity" aerobic exercise, which is perfect for warming up your muscles or cooling them down from an intense aerobic workout. It's also a safe zone for exercisers who want to preserve their muscle size, but who are looking to exercise the heart for health reasons.

Sixty to 70 percent of your MHR: This zone is the most popular, mostly because this "medium-intensity" level of cardiovascular exercise pushes your muscles at a level that's optimal for burning excess body fat.

Seventy to 80 percent of your MHR: Pushing yourself at this "high-intensity" pace can be the solution for several different types of goals. It's perfect for time-starved exercisers looking to burn fat with what few minutes they may have to spare. Maintaining your pulse at 70 to 80 percent of your MHR not only burns calories but also taxes your heart and lungs even further. Pushing your aerobic boundaries can increase your endurance and decrease your risk of cardiovascular diseases. However, the high caloric expenditure makes this pace an unwise choice for anyone looking to achieve maximum size and strength with their muscles.

Eighty percent of your MHR or higher: Sure, it's possible to go higher than 80 percent. But if you're reading this book, odds are you're looking to shape your body, not push it past its own physical capabilities. This level of intensity is optimal for improving your maximum VO_2 levels—the highest amount of oxygen your body can take in during exercise. But it's usually reserved for endurance athletes who are looking to train for a specific sport-related goal.

Trying to elevate your pulse to this level of intensity may sound like a bright idea for burning even *more* calories. However, this type of intensity can be too stressful for many average exercisers, and it can increase your risk of injury, leaving your body regretful—instead of grateful—that you tried it.

One Last Thing Before You Start . . .

This book provides 120 different workouts that you can use in any situation, but that doesn't mean you *only* have to use them when it's absolutely necessary!

Know this: Maintenance doesn't always help to preserve things. If you're the type of person who

can consistently put in 3 days a week and 45 minutes per workout, that doesn't mean you should just keep using your prescribed workout over and over again.

As I said earlier in this book, your muscles adapt to any exercise within five or six workouts,

> YOUR BODY STARTS TO BURN FEWER CALORIES AND USE FEWER MUSCLE FIBERS DURING YOUR WORKOUTS, LEAVING YOU WITH LESS-SATISFYING OVERALL RESULTS FOR ALL YOUR HARD WORK. BREAKING THIS VICIOUS CYCLE REQUIRES ONLY A FEW MODIFICATIONS TO YOUR EXERCISE ROUTINES.

so customizing your workout every few weeks can keep your heart and other muscles challenged enough to change for the better. Most people get stuck in a holding pattern because they're too scared to stray from a routine that's worked in the past. The truth is, sticking with what works *could be holding you back.*

Whether your goal is to burn fat, build a stronger chest, or bulk up all over, each of these "exercise achievements" is just a biological response to whatever physical stress your exercise routine has placed on your muscles. These adaptations eventually stop as your body begins to figure out more energy-efficient ways of dealing with the stress. The result? Your body starts to burn fewer calories and use fewer muscle fibers during your workouts, and this leaves you with less-satisfying overall results for all your hard work.

Breaking this vicious cycle requires only a few modifications to your exercise routines. And now

ONE FINAL THING BEFORE YOU BEGIN . . .

Before you try out any—or hopefully all—of the workouts you're about to learn in the next few chapters of this book, there's something you need to know. The positive results we want and expect from exercise—losing body fat, building muscle, being able to work out longer, being able to lift heavier and heavier amounts of weight, and so forth—don't always come one after another at the same, ever-improving pace. You will start seeing a leaner, stronger, fat-free physique faster than you ever expected, but there will be some days when you may feel as if your body has failed you.

Throughout the next few weeks, months, years, and decades of using this book to change your body—and your life—for the better, I want you to make me a promise. If you ever find yourself wondering why some days you outperform yourself with your exercise while on others you can't seem to work out as hard as you usually do, then find your way back to this section.

It might not be the workout that's failing you . . . it could be *you* that's failing the workout!

In chapter 2, you were shown how overtraining your muscles can make them weaker if you're not careful. There are, however, other factors that also affect your performance on an individual day-to-day basis. Dietary changes, sleeping patterns, and everyday stress can all play a small part in affecting your exercise each day, which is something most people aren't aware of. The moment they see their performance starting to slip—even if for just a few days—they assume that

their exercise plan is no longer effective. That's why many people quit the right routine for them way sooner than they should, never achieving the results that were waiting for them if they had just stuck with the exercise plan.

Being aware of any "outside interference" that might be hampering your performance can keep you from quitting the right exercise plan too soon. To make it easy for you to evaluate your day, just ask yourself the following eight questions. If you find yourself answering yes to any of them, it could explain why your body is saying no to giving you 100 percent.

1. Did you deal with any amount of stress at work or home today?

2. Did you get less than 8 hours of sleep last night?

3. Did you drink less than 64 ounces of water, juice, or milk today?

4. Did you eat less than five servings of fruits or vegetables today?

5. Did you eat more than 60 grams of fat today?

6. Did you eat less than 8 ounces of protein (fish, chicken, or lean meat) today?

7. Did you drink alcohol today?

8. Have you been using the same exact workout for more than 2 months?

that you have this book, the "mods" you need are right at your fingertips.

If an ever-changing schedule forces you to adjust your workouts from week to week, you'll have no choice but to use a variety of the workouts in this book, which will automatically mix things up for your muscles so they're constantly challenged.

But if every week for you is the same old routine, then do yourself—and your body—a favor. If you usually exercise 4 days a week, try 5—or 3—every once in a while. If you typically work out for 45 minutes, give 60 minutes a shot. Or scale your routine back to 20 minutes—or 10 minutes—just to see what it feels like.

Luckily, each of the 48 "anytime" exercises that we'll cover in chapter 4 is designed to be performed in several different ways, using different types of equipment. That means that if you decide to stick with, let's say, the same 3-day-a-week workout plan that uses the same eight exercises week after week, all you have to do to make the routine fresh enough for your muscles is try a variation or two of each exercise every few weeks.

Just replacing *one* key anytime exercise with any of its variations can feel different enough to make your body think it's trying something entirely new. That, in itself, can rejuvenate your workouts.

CHAPTER 4

Your 48 "Anytime" Exercises

You know how many days in the week you have to work out. You know how much time each day you have to work out. You even know what type of results-specific workout you want to put your body through. Now, all that's left is picking the best moves to help you accomplish your goals.

Introducing . . . the 48 "anytime" exercises!

Why "anytime"? Because no matter where you are, no matter who you are, these are the only exercises you'll ever need to use, regardless of your current exercise goals.

Don't have a degree in exercise physiology? Don't worry, you won't need one. Unlike other fitness books that expect you to find exercises according to which body part they work, we've placed the moves in alphabetical order so you can find them instantly. Want to make sure you're using the right exercise for the right muscle group? Just refer to "What's It Working?" directly below the exercise name, to give you peace of mind. Otherwise, just do whatever each routine instructs you to do and you'll get the best full-body workout you can in whatever time you have to give.

To keep you exercising no matter what the circumstances, each of the 48 moves gives you a few alternatives to choose from.

GET IT RIGHT FOR MORE RESULTS!

The first version of each exercise that's mentioned should always be the first version you choose—unless you're ready for a new challenge or can't do the exercise because you lack the right equipment. We'll get to those situations in a minute.

If you've ever resented anyone for their physique, you can stop now. The bodies that have earned your exercise envy may not be more committed to working out than you are, it's just that they're smarter when it comes to *how* they work out.

Now it's your turn.

The secret to getting in great shape isn't how much time you spend exercising, it's taking the time to exercise properly. One simple slip in form can turn a useful exercise into a useless one that neglects the problem zones you're trying to reach, while stressing overworked areas you would rather avoid.

To get the most from each of the 48 anytime exercises, you have to do each one correctly from the start. Follow the instructions given in each of these sections and your muscles will always make the most of every move.

THE SECRET TO GETTING IN GREAT SHAPE ISN'T HOW MUCH TIME YOU SPEND EXERCISING, IT'S TAKING THE TIME TO EXERCISE PROPERLY. ONE SIMPLE SLIP IN FORM CAN TURN A USEFUL EXERCISE INTO A USELESS ONE.

GOT ADDITIONAL EQUIPMENT?

Having a gym membership—or a well-stocked home gym—means having an array of unique exercise tools, machines, and perhaps a training partner or two at your disposal. That gives your muscles even more options. Trying these variations of the 48 anytime exercises can help you burn more calories, build more lean muscle, and achieve more results down the road.

GOT NOTHING TO USE?

The problem with most exercise books is that, while they tell you about a wide variety of exercises you should do, they forget that sometimes even the basics can be impossible to pull off—especially if you don't have access to much exercise equipment. Maybe the hotel you're staying at is lucky to have running water. Or maybe you're nervous about investing money in exercise equipment just yet. That's when this option can save your workout.

SO WHAT EXACTLY *IS* A "LIGHT WEIGHT," ANYWAY?

You may notice that some "anytime" exercises ask you to grab a "light" dumbbell, barbell, or medicine ball. Since what may be less heavy for some people may be too heavy for others, it's wise to do a little pre-exercise planning. The very first time you perform an exercise, start with the bare minimum in terms of poundage, then increase the weight with each set until you find a poundage that lets you do the exercise within the required amount of repetitions. For example, if an anytime exercise requires . . .

. . . *a light dumbbell (or two):* Start with a 1-pound dumbbell(s). The smallest dumbbells run about a pound and typically increase in increments of 1 to 2½ pounds until they reach 25 pounds—after that, they usually get heavier in 5-pound increments.

. . . *a light barbell:* Start by using just the weight of the bar, with no weights added. A standard weight bar—which can range from 5 to 7 feet in length—weighs an average of 13 to 20 pounds, depending on the length and style. A 7-foot Olympic bar weighs around 45 pounds. (A shorter, 5-foot Olympic bar is about 30 pounds.) Once the bar feels too light, you can start adding 2½-pound weight plates on both ends, increasing the weight in increments of 5 pounds.

. . . *a light medicine ball:* Start with the lightest ball you can find, which is around 2 to 2.2 pounds. Once you feel strong enough to try more weight than that, keep in mind that medicine balls typically increase in 2-pound increments (4 to 4.4 pounds, 6 to 6.6 pounds, etc.).

THE ANYTIME EXERCISES CHECKLIST

#1: Bench press

#2: Bent-over reverse raise

#3: Bent-over row

#4: Biceps curl

#5: Chest fly

#6: Close-grip pulldown

#7: Crunch

#8: Deadlift

#9: Decline press

#10: Dip

#11: Front raise

#12: Front squat

#13: Good morning

#14: Hammer curl

#15: Incline fly

#16: Incline press

#17: Kickback

#18: Lateral raise

#19: Lat pulldown

#20: Leg curl

#21: Leg extension

#22: Lunge

#23: Lying triceps press

#24: One-arm row

#25: One-arm triceps extension

#26: Power clean

#27: Preacher curl

#28: Pullover

#29: Push press

#30: Reverse crunch

#31: Reverse curl

#32: Reverse lunge

#33: Seated calf raise

#34: Seated shoulder press

#35: Seated triceps extension

#36: Shrug

#37: Side lunge

#38: Side raise

#39: Squat

#40: Standing calf raise

#41: Triceps pushdown

#42: Twisting crunch

#43: Twisting leg thrust

#44: Twisting toe touch

#45: Upright row

#46: V-up with a twist

#47: Wrist curl

#48: Wrist extension

To perform the bare-bones versions of the anytime exercises, the only equipment that you will ever need to invest in is a basic set of dumbbells. If you don't see a bare-bones version of an exercise in this chapter, that means the original version already requires you to use nothing more than a set of dumbbells—or your own body weight.

Now that you have the time and the right tools, you're ready to take on exercise any day of the week, week by week, for the rest of your life!

Anytime Exercise #1: BENCH PRESS

WHAT'S IT WORKING? Your chest, anterior deltoids, and triceps

Get it right for more results!

Lie faceup on an exercise bench with your knees bent and your feet flat on the floor. Grab a dumbbell in each hand and position them along the sides of your chest. (Your elbows should be bent at a 90-degree angle and your palms turned toward your knees.) Push the weights upward until your arms are fully extended above your chest, elbows unlocked. Slowly lower the weights back along the sides of your chest, and repeat.

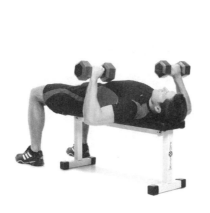 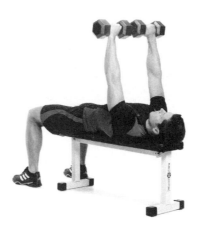

Got additional equipment?

Lie on an exercise bench and grab a barbell with your hands slightly wider than shoulder width apart. Place your feet flat on the floor, lift the bar off the rack, and hold it straight above your chest, elbows unlocked. (Your arms should be perpendicular to the floor.) Slowly lower the bar until it touches your chest, press the weight back up until your arms are straight once more, and repeat.

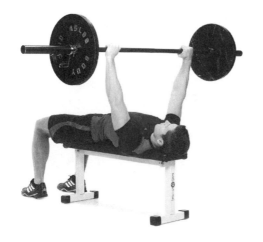 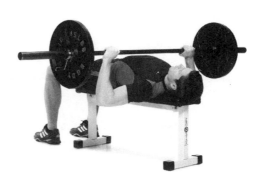

Got nothing to use?

Do a pushup by placing your hands flat on the floor (shoulder width apart) with your arms straight and elbows unlocked. Straighten your legs behind you, drawing your feet together. Rise up on your toes so the top of the balls of your feet are touching the floor. Your body should be one straight line from your heels to your head, your eyes focused straight down at the ground. Without moving your head, slowly lower yourself until your upper arms are parallel to the ground. Pause, slowly push yourself back up, and repeat.

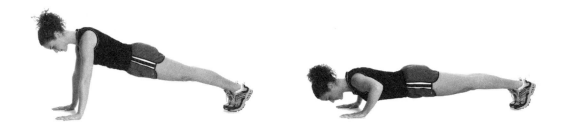

Anytime Exercise #2: BENT-OVER REVERSE RAISE

WHAT'S IT WORKING? Your posterior deltoids and middle trapezius

Get it right for more results!

Sit on the end of an exercise bench with a light weight in each hand. Your arms should hang straight down at your sides, palms facing each other. Bending at the waist, lean forward so your chest comes down a few inches from your thighs. Keeping your arms straight, slowly raise the weights up behind you until they are parallel to the floor. Pause, then slowly lower your arms so that the weights are again hanging toward the floor, and repeat.

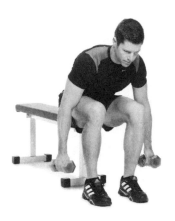 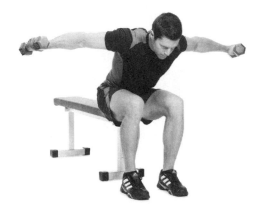

Got additional equipment?

This variation requires a cable crossover machine with two low pulley stations. Stand between the two cable towers with your feet about shoulder width apart. Cross your hands in front of you, lean down, and grab a pulley in each hand—your left hand will be holding the right cable pulley and your right hand will be holding the left cable pulley. With your knees slightly bent and your back straight, lean forward until your torso is parallel to the floor. Your arms should be hanging below you with your hands crossed over each other. With your elbows slightly bent, slowly raise your arms out to your sides until they are parallel to the floor. Pause, slowly lower your arms back down below your chest, and repeat.

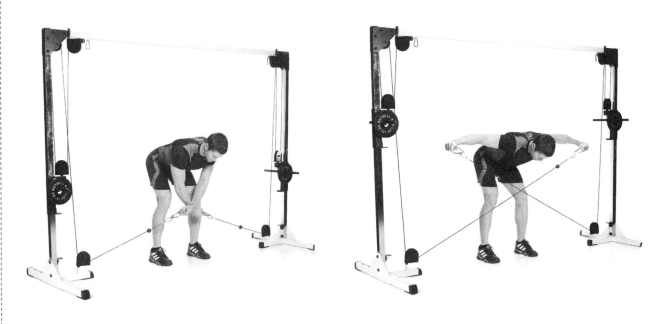

Anytime Exercise #3: BENT-OVER ROW

WHAT'S IT WORKING? Your latissimus dorsi, trapezius, posterior deltoids, and biceps

Get it right for more results!

Place a barbell on the floor in front of you and stand behind it with your feet shoulder width apart, knees slightly bent. Reach down and grab the bar overhand, hands slightly wider than shoulder width apart. Lift the barbell off the floor until your torso is parallel to the floor. (Your arms should be extended straight below you.) Keeping your back and legs locked in this position, slowly pull the bar up until it touches the bottom of your chest. Pause, slowly lower the bar back down, and repeat.

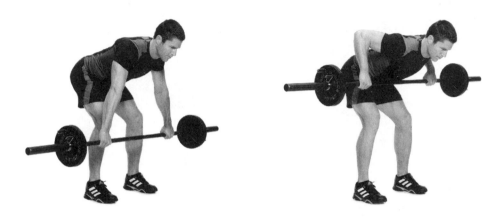

Got additional equipment?

Attach a lat-pulldown bar to a low cable rowing machine. Sit on the floor, bend forward at the waist, and grab the bar with your hands toward the ends. (They should be spaced slightly wider than shoulder width apart.) Next, lean back into an upright position. (Your back should end up perpendicular to the floor; leaning back any farther will put unnecessary stress on your lower back.) Holding this position, slowly pull the bar to your midsection. Allow the bar to pull your arms back out in front of you, until you're back in the starting position, and repeat.

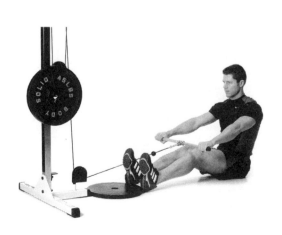 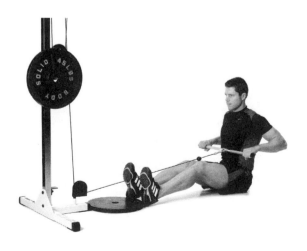

Got nothing to use?

Stand straight with a light dumbbell in each hand, arms down at your sides. Bend forward at the waist until your back is almost parallel to the floor. Your legs should be straight but unlocked; your arms should hang straight down with palms facing each other. While keeping your arms close to your torso, raise both dumbbells straight up until they touch the sides of your chest. Pause, slowly lower the weights until your arms are straight once more, and repeat.

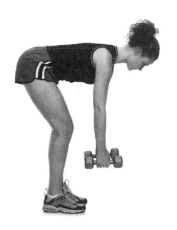 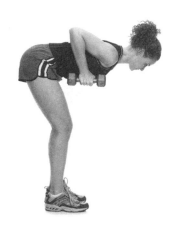

Anytime Exercise #4: BICEPS CURL

WHAT'S IT WORKING? Your biceps and forearms

Get it right for more results!

Stand holding a barbell with an underhand grip, your hands shoulder width apart. Your arms should hang straight so that the bar touches the fronts of your thighs. Keeping your elbows tucked into your sides, slowly curl the bar up until it reaches your chest. Pause, slowly lower the bar back down, and repeat.

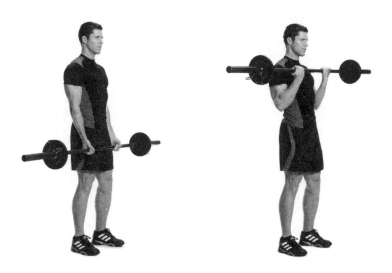

Got additional equipment?

Attach a straight bar to a low cable pulley and stand facing the weight stack about 1 to 2 feet away. Grab the bar with an underhand grip—palms facing up—with your hands about shoulder width apart. With your elbows fixed at your sides, slowly curl the bar up until it's just below your chin. Pause, lower the bar back down in front of you, and repeat.

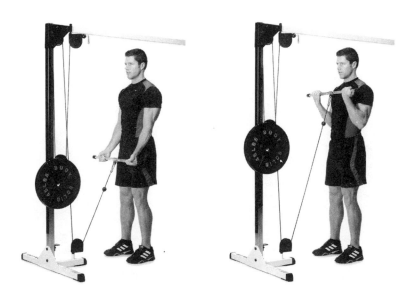

Got nothing to use?

Stand holding a dumbbell in each hand, with your arms hanging at your sides and your palms facing out in front of you. Keeping your back straight, slowly curl the weights up—your palms should end up facing the fronts of your shoulders. Slowly lower the weights back down, and repeat.

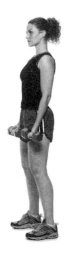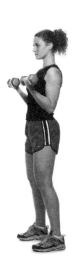

Anytime Exercise #5: CHEST FLY

WHAT'S IT WORKING? Your chest, shoulders, and the serratus anterior muscles (along the rib cage)

Get it right for more results!

Lie on your back on a flat exercise bench with a dumbbell in each hand. Bend your knees so that your feet are flat on the floor. Raise your arms straight above your chest, your palms facing each other and your elbows slightly bent. Slowly lower the dumbbells in an arc so that your hands end up out to your sides with your elbows bent about 90 degrees. Slowly raise the weights, again following the same arc, until the weights are together directly above your chest, and repeat.

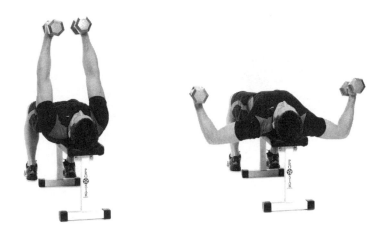

Got additional equipment?

Place an exercise bench between two cable towers. Lie faceup on the bench with your knees bent and your feet flat on the floor. Hold a cable handle in each hand, and extend your arms straight up above your shoulders, palms facing each other. Bend your elbows slightly, then slowly lower your arms in an arc out to your sides as far as it is comfortable. Bring your arms back to the starting position, keeping the same semicircular arc throughout the movement, and repeat.

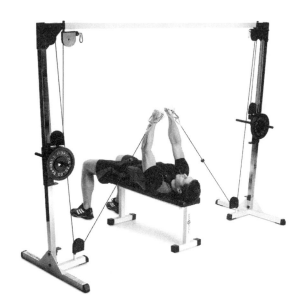
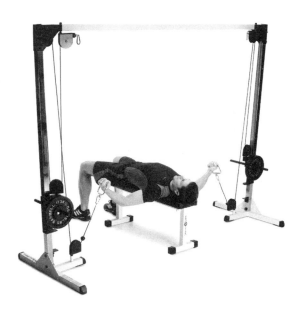

Anytime Exercise #6: CLOSE-GRIP PULLDOWN

WHAT'S IT WORKING? Your latissimus dorsi

Get it right for more results!

Sit at a lat-pulldown station—or on a bench with a high-pulley attachment—and grab the bar with an underhand grip, your hands spaced about 6 inches apart and your palms facing toward you. Slowly pull the bar down to the front of your chest. Resist the weight as you let the bar raise your hands back above your head, and repeat.

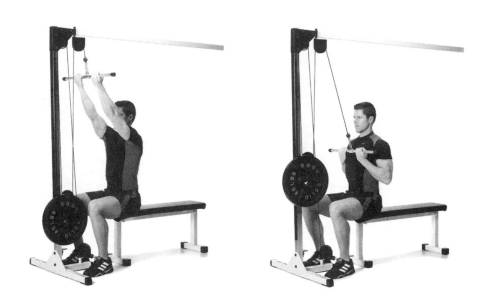

Got additional equipment?

Angle an incline exercise bench between 30 and 40 degrees, then sit on it backward. Lean all the way forward, resting your chest and face flat on the bench. Grab a light dumbbell in each hand, letting your arms hang straight down with your palms facing each other. Keeping your upper arms close to your body, slowly draw the weights up to the sides of your chest until your elbows are in line with your back. Slowly lower the weights back down to the floor, and repeat.

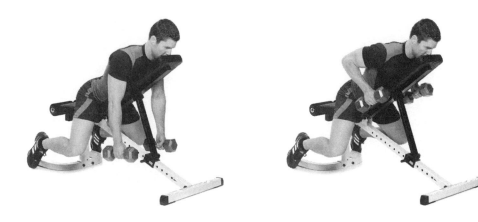

Got nothing to use?

Grab the pullup bar with an underhand grip and with your hands spaced 6 to 12 inches apart, your palms facing back. Hang from the bar so that your arms are straight, then slowly pull yourself up until the bar is directly under your chin. Squeeze your back muscles at the top, slowly lower yourself back down until your arms are straight once again, and repeat.

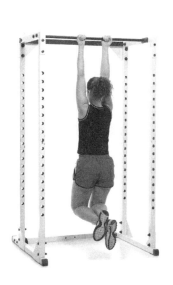
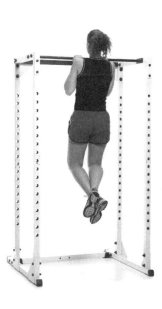

Anytime Exercise #7: CRUNCH

WHAT'S IT WORKING? Your upper rectus abdominis

Get it right for more results!

Sit on top of a stability ball with your legs in front of you and your feet flat on the floor. Slowly lean back and roll yourself down the ball until just your head, shoulders, and back are touching it—your back should shape itself to the curve of the ball. Touch your hands lightly alongside your ears, and you're ready to begin. Keeping your balance, slowly lift your head, arms, and upper back off the ball. Lower back down, and repeat.

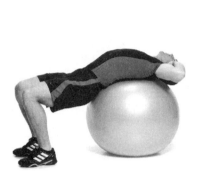 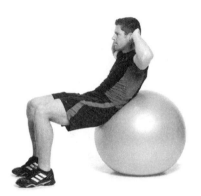

Got additional equipment?

Get on your knees with your back toward a high cable pulley with a rope attachment, and grab both ends of the rope. Draw your hands either down by the sides of your ears (palms facing in) or just down below your chin (palms touching the top of your chest). Keeping your hands locked in place, bend at the waist and slowly curl yourself down as far as you comfortably can. Reverse the motion, bringing yourself back up into the starting position, and repeat.

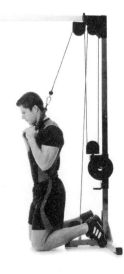 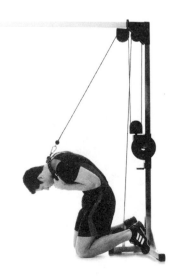

Got nothing to use?

Lie flat on the floor with your knees bent, feet shoulder width apart. Place your hands along the sides of your head so that they're lightly touching behind your ears. As you begin to exhale, slowly curl your head and torso toward your knees until your shoulder blades are off the floor, keeping your feet flat and your hands alongside your head. Imagine that you're drawing your ribs to your hips, as if your midsection were an accordion. Pause, lower yourself back down, and repeat.

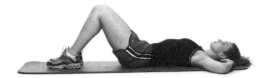 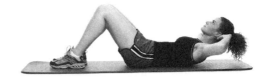

Anytime Exercise #8: DEADLIFT

WHAT'S IT WORKING? Your gluteal muscles, hamstrings, quadriceps, latissimus dorsi, trapezius, erector spinae, forearms, obliques, and abdominals

Get it right for more results!

Stand facing a barbell, with the bar over your toes. Bend your knees and grasp the bar with an alternating grip (one underhand; one overhand). Your feet should be spaced shoulder width apart, your hands slightly wider. Keeping your head and back straight, slowly stand up, keeping the bar close to your body as you lift, until your legs are straight but your knees aren't locked. Pause for a second, slowly lower the bar back down to the floor, and repeat.

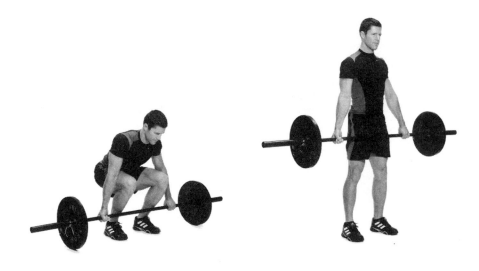

Got additional equipment?

Instead of starting with the bar on the floor, position the bar off the floor by placing the weight on a power rack with the pins set low. The weight plates should be raised about 12 to 18 inches off the floor. Performing the deadlift from this position eliminates the bottom portion of the exercise, making it easier to use heavier amounts of weight in the move for more results.

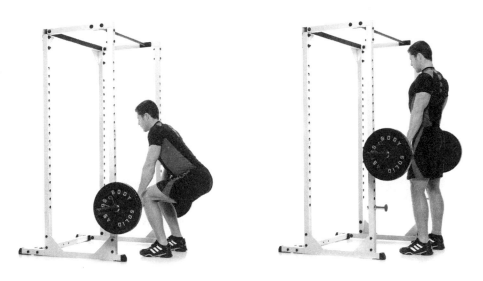

Got nothing to use?

Stand with your feet shoulder width apart and place a dumbbell just outside of each foot. Bend your knees and grab the dumbbells with your palms facing in. Keeping your head up and your back straight, slowly stand up until your legs are straight but your knees aren't locked. Keep the weights close to your body as you lift. Pause, slowly lower the weights back down to the floor, and repeat.

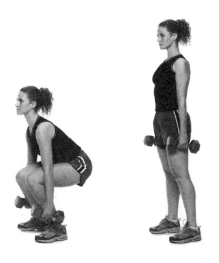

Anytime Exercise #9: DECLINE PRESS

WHAT'S IT WORKING? Your lower pectoral muscles, shoulders, and triceps

Get it right for more results!

Lie back on a decline bench with your head at the low end and your feet either flat or secured at the high end. Grab a pair of dumbbells and position them above your head with your arms extended straight up, perpendicular to the floor, palms facing your knees. Slowly lower the dumbbells down to the outer edges of your chest, just below your nipples. Press them back up above your chest, keeping your elbows unlocked at the top, and repeat.

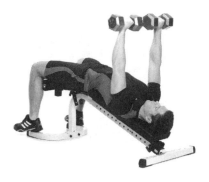 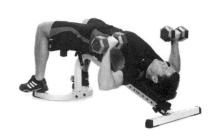

Got additional equipment?

Lie on a decline bench and grab a barbell in an overhand grip with your hands slightly wider than shoulder width apart. Hold the bar straight above your chest, with your elbows unlocked. (Your arms should be perpendicular to the floor.) Slowly lower the bar until it touches your chest, press the weight back up until your arms are straight once more, and repeat.

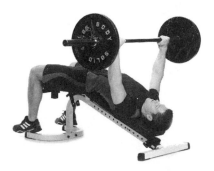 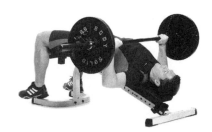

Got nothing to use?

Kneel on the floor facing a staircase. Place your hands flat on the second step, about shoulder width apart, and extend your legs behind you. Lower yourself down by bending your elbows, keeping your knees locked and your legs and back straight. Press back up to the starting position, and repeat.

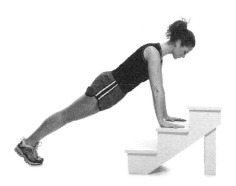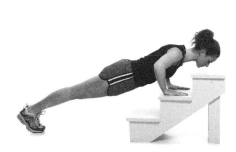

Anytime Exercise #10: DIP

WHAT'S IT WORKING? Your triceps and pectoral muscles

Get it right for more results!

Stand on a box in front of a set of parallel bars, and grab the bars with your arms straight. Your palms should face in, and your knuckles should point down toward the floor. Keep your elbows close to your sides but not locked, and step off the box so that you're supporting your weight with your arms. Bend your knees so that your feet won't hit the box as you lower yourself. Slowly lower yourself until your upper arms are parallel to the floor. Press yourself back up until your arms are once again straight with elbows unlocked, and repeat.

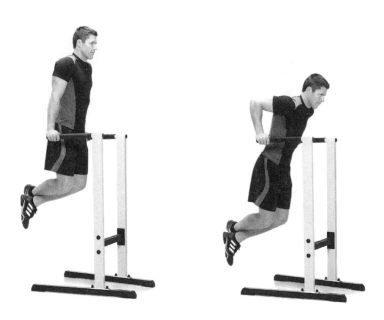

Got additional equipment?

Strap on a dip belt and add a few weight plates (approximately 20 percent of your body weight) to start. Stand on the box and grab the set of parallel dip bars with your arms straight and your palms facing in. Keep your elbows close to your sides and your legs bent as you slowly lower yourself down until your upper arms are parallel to the floor (this should take about 4 seconds). Continue to support your weight in this lowered position as you step back onto the box. Stand back into position so that your arms are once again straight, elbows unlocked, and repeat.

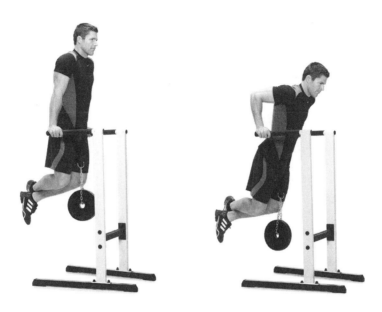

Got nothing to use?

Place two high, sturdy chairs next to each other and kneel between them. Place one hand on the seat of each chair near your waist, positioning them so that your fingers are pointing straight ahead of you, elbows pointing back. With your hands kept in place and your knees bent, slowly straighten your arms to raise yourself off the floor. (Keep your elbows close to your sides and unlocked.) Slowly bend your arms and lower yourself down until your knees almost touch the floor, and repeat.

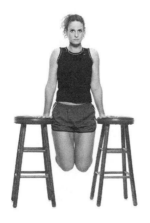
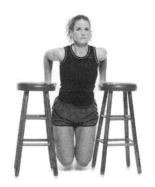

Anytime Exercise #11: FRONT RAISE

WHAT'S IT WORKING? Your anterior deltoids

Get it right for more results!

Stand straight with your feet 18 to 24 inches apart, holding a barbell in front of you, with your arms down and your palms facing your thighs. Your hands should be about shoulder width apart with your fingers resting on your thighs. Keeping your back and arms straight, slowly raise the bar in front of you until your arms are parallel to the floor. Pause, slowly lower the bar until your hands almost touch your thighs, and repeat.

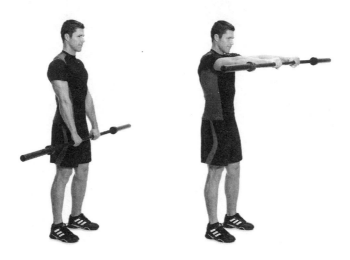

Got additional equipment?

Stand with your back to a low pulley station, with the handle in your right hand, your palm facing behind you. Keeping your back and arms straight, slowly raise your right arm straight up in front of you until it's parallel to the floor. Pause, then slowly lower the handle straight down until your right arm is alongside your body once more. Repeat for 1 set, then perform the exercise again with your left arm.

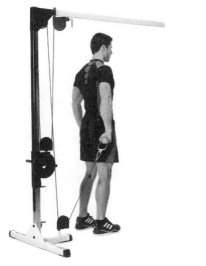 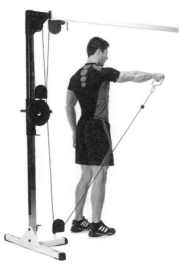

Got nothing to use?

Stand straight with your feet about 12 inches apart, holding a light dumbbell in each hand. Your arms should be at your sides and slightly forward, your palms facing your thighs. Keeping your arms straight, slowly raise the weights in front of you until they are parallel to the floor, palms facing down. Pause, slowly lower your arms back down, and repeat.

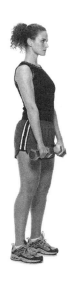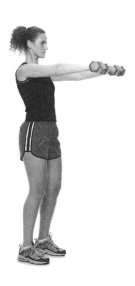

Anytime Exercise #12: FRONT SQUAT

WHAT'S IT WORKING? Your quadriceps and gluteal muscles

Get it right for more results!

Stand holding a pair of dumbbells, with your feet shoulder width apart and your knees unlocked. Bring the weights up in front of your body and rest the end of each dumbbell on the top of each shoulder—your palms should be facing each other with your elbows pointing out. Slowly squat down until your thighs are parallel to the floor. Pause, push yourself back into a standing position, and repeat.

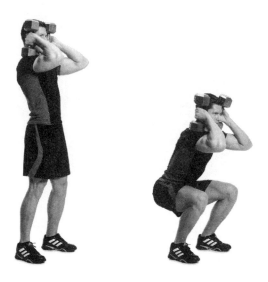

Got additional equipment?

Place a barbell at chest height on a squat rack and stand facing it. With your legs shoulder width apart and your feet pointing straight ahead, step in close to the barbell so that the bar touches your upper chest, then reach under the barbell with both arms. Cross your arms over the bar and grab it with your palms facing down toward your chest, your hands close together. Lift the weight, resting the bar across the top of your chest. (This crossed-arm position gives you a more secure grip.) With your back straight, squat down until your thighs are almost parallel to the floor. Pause, push yourself back into a standing position, and repeat.

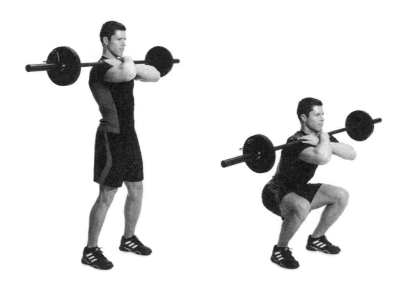

Anytime Exercise #13: GOOD MORNING

WHAT'S IT WORKING? Your hamstrings, gluteal muscles, and lower back

Get it right for more results!

Stand with your feet hip width apart and rest a light barbell comfortably across your shoulders, holding it with palms facing forward. Keeping your back flat and your head in line with your spine, slowly bend forward at the waist until your torso is almost parallel to the floor. Reverse the motion until you're back in a standing position, and repeat.

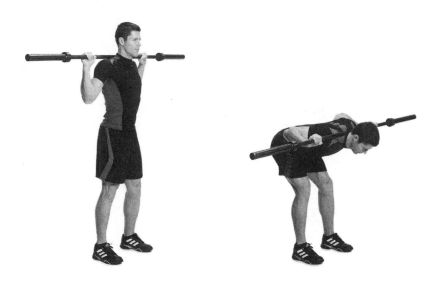

Got additional equipment?

This exercise requires a hyperextension bench, commonly found at most gyms. A hyper-extension bench has a wide horizontal pad in front, a thin pad in back, and two handles on the sides.

Step between the pads, hold on to the handles for support, and lean forward so that your thighs rest on the wide pad and your legs tuck underneath the thin pads. Lock your hands behind your head and bend forward at the waist until your upper body is almost perpendicular to the floor. (This is the starting position.) Slowly raise your torso until it's slightly higher than parallel with the floor. Return to the starting position, and repeat.

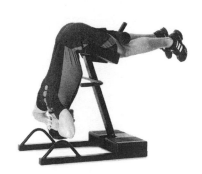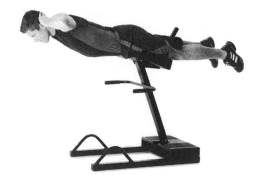

Got nothing to use?

Lie on your stomach with your arms pointing straight in front of you—as if you were flying. Slowly raise your arms, chest, head, and legs off the floor simultaneously and hold for a count of two. Lower yourself back down, and repeat.

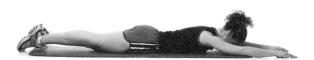 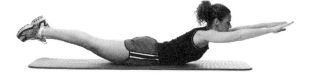

Anytime Exercise #14: HAMMER CURL

WHAT'S IT WORKING? Your biceps and forearms

Get it right for more results!

Stand straight with a dumbbell in each hand, your arms at your sides. Your palms should be facing in toward your thighs. Keeping your back straight, slowly curl both dumbbells toward your shoulders, keeping your wrists from turning as you go. Your thumbs should be pointing toward your shoulders at the top of the move. Slowly lower the weights back down until your arms are straight, and repeat.

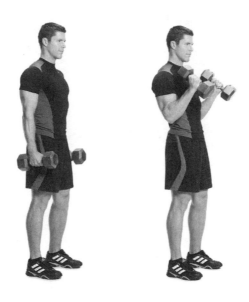

Got additional equipment?

Attach a rope to a low cable pulley and stand facing the weight stack, about 1 to 2 feet away. Grab the rope with both hands and space them about shoulder width apart, palms facing each other. With your elbows tucked into your sides, slowly curl your fists up until they are directly in front of your chest. Pause, lower your hands back down in front of you, and repeat.

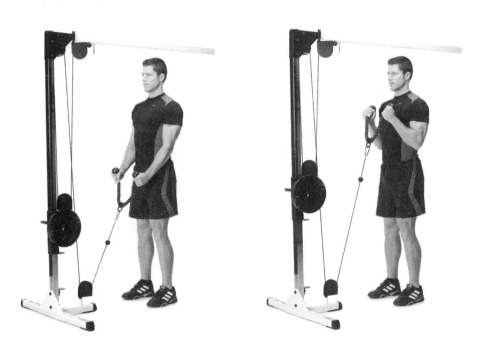

Anytime Exercise #15: INCLINE FLY

WHAT'S IT WORKING? Your upper pectorals

Get it right for more results!

Grab a pair of light dumbbells and lie on an incline exercise bench, with your feet flat on the floor. Hold the weights directly over your chest, with your elbows slightly bent and your palms facing in toward each other. In a semicircular arcing motion, slowly lower the weights out to your sides until your upper arms are parallel to the floor. Raise the dumbbells back up in an arcing motion until they are back above your chest, and repeat.

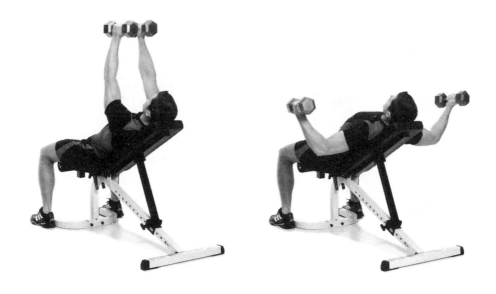

Got additional equipment?

Place an incline exercise bench between two low pulleys. Lie back on the bench, then reach to both sides and take a handle in each hand. Bring them together at arm's length above your chest, your palms facing each other. With your elbows slightly bent, slowly lower your hands out to your sides in an arc. Slowly bring your hands back up above you, and repeat.

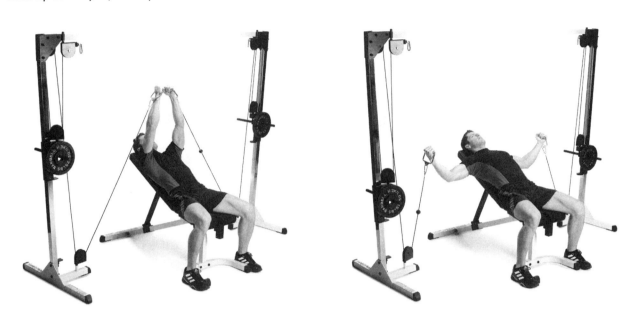

Anytime Exercise #16: INCLINE PRESS

WHAT'S IT WORKING? Your upper pectorals

Get it right for more results!

Lie back on an incline exercise bench with a dumbbell in each hand. Raise the weights so that they rest along the outside of your chest, with your palms facing forward. Slowly press the dumbbells straight up above your chest, touching them together at the top. (Avoid locking your elbows; this will only take tension off your chest muscles.) Slowly lower the weights back down along the sides of your chest, and repeat.

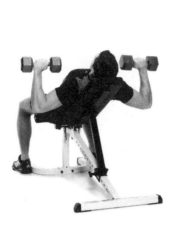
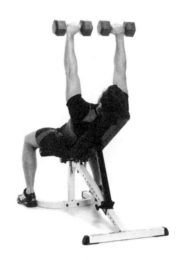

Got additional equipment?

Position yourself on an incline exercise bench, and grab the bar above you so that your hands are slightly wider than shoulder width apart, and your palms are facing forward. Have a spotter help you lift the weight from the rack, then position the bar directly above your chest. Slowly lower the bar down until it lightly touches the top portion of your chest, press the weight back above you, and repeat.

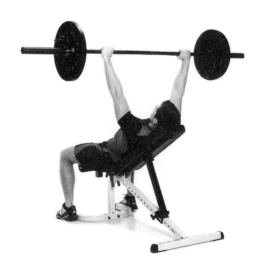
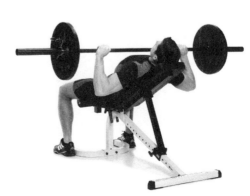

Got nothing to use?

Stand with your back to a staircase, then kneel down and place your hands flat on the floor, shoulder width apart. Place your feet up on the second step of the staircase and straighten your body into the classic pushup position. Lower yourself down until your upper arms are parallel to the floor, then press yourself back up, and repeat.

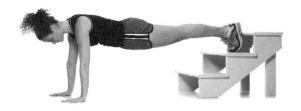 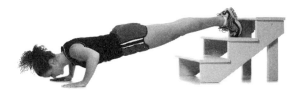

Anytime Exercise #17: KICKBACK

WHAT'S IT WORKING? Your triceps

Get it right for more results!

Stand with your left side to the exercise bench and a light dumbbell in your right hand. Rest your left hand and knee on the bench, bend at the waist, and let your right arm hang down toward the floor, your palm facing in toward the bench. Slowly draw the weight up close to your body until your upper arm is parallel to the floor. Your right arm should resemble a right angle, with the weight hanging down to the floor. Keeping your upper arm stationary, slowly straighten your right arm out behind you. Pause, then bend your elbow to lower the weight back down, and repeat. At the end of the set, switch positions to work your left arm.

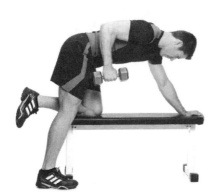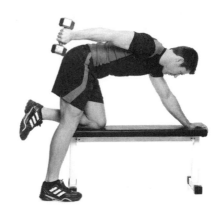

Got additional equipment?

Place an exercise bench lengthwise in front of a low cable station, and attach a rope to the end of the pulley. Stand facing the station, grab one end of the rope with your left hand, and position yourself on the left side of the bench. Bend at the waist and rest your right hand and knee on the bench. Pull your left arm up so that your upper arm is close to your side and parallel to the floor, your palm facing in. Holding this position, slowly extend your left arm straight behind you. Pause, reverse the motion, and repeat. At the end of the set, switch positions to work your right arm.

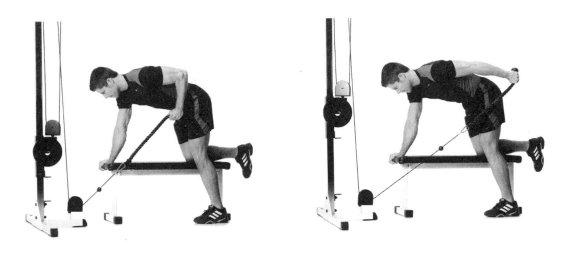

Anytime Exercise #18: LATERAL RAISE

WHAT'S IT WORKING? Your medial deltoids and upper trapezius

Get it right for more results!

Stand straight with your feet shoulder width apart and hold a light dumbbell in each hand. Your arms should hang down and your palms should face in toward each other. Keeping your arms straight, slowly raise them out to your sides until they're parallel to the floor. (You'll look like the letter T.) Pause at the top of the movement for a second, then slowly lower your arms back down to your sides, and repeat.

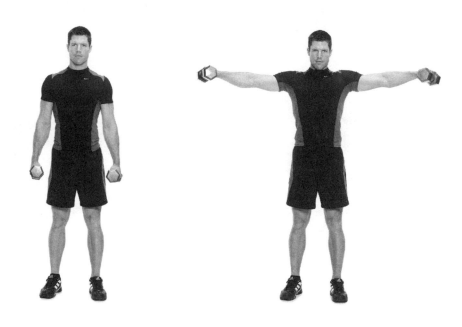

Got additional equipment?

Stand between the two cable towers of a cable crossover machine with your feet about shoulder width apart. Cross your arms in front of you, lean down and grab a low pulley handle in each hand, then return to a standing position. Your left hand will be holding the right-side cable and your right hand will be holding the left-side cable, with wrists crossed in front of your waist. With your elbows slightly bent and your back straight, slowly pull both handles upward and out to the sides of your body until your arms are parallel to the floor. (You'll look like the letter T.) Pause at the top of the movement for a second, slowly lower your hands to the starting position, and repeat.

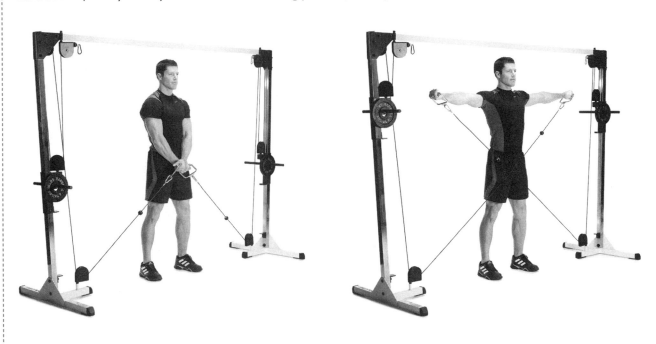

Anytime Exercise #19: LAT PULLDOWN

WHAT'S IT WORKING? Your latissimus dorsi, middle and upper trapezius, and biceps

Get it right for more results!

Sit at a lat-pulldown station—or on a bench with a high-pulley attachment—and grab the bar overhead with an overhand grip, your hands slightly wider than shoulder width apart. Keeping your head and back straight, slowly pull the bar down until it touches just above your chest. Slowly let the bar rise above your head—resisting the weight as you go—until your arms are straight again, elbows unlocked, and repeat.

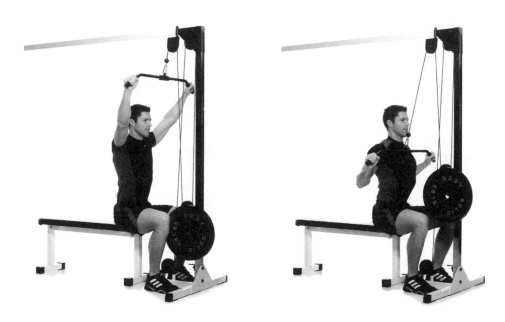

Got additional equipment?

This one takes a little tinkering, but it's well worth it. Attach a strap to both sides of a lat-pulldown bar, spacing the straps about 3 feet apart from each other. Slip your hands through the straps so that your palms face each other. Sit down and let your arms be pulled above your head. Slowly pull your hands down to the sides of your shoulders. Let the bar rise slowly back to the starting position, and repeat.

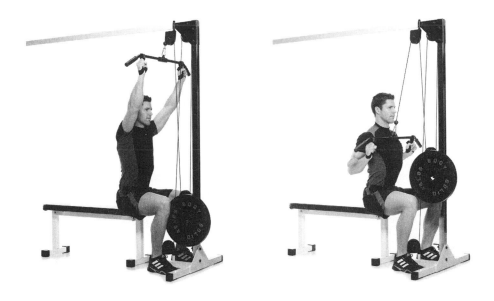

Got nothing to use?

Grab a chinup bar with your hands slightly wider than shoulder width apart, your palms facing away from you. Let yourself hang with your arms straight, elbows un-locked. Slowly pull yourself up until the bar is directly under your chin, then lower yourself back down, and repeat.

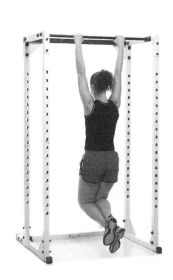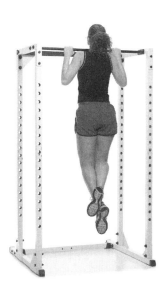

Anytime Exercise #20: LEG CURL

WHAT'S IT WORKING? Your hamstrings and gluteal muscles

Get it right for more results!

For this exercise, you'll need an exercise bench with a leg curl attachment at the end.

Lie facedown on the bench, tucking your ankles underneath the pads. Your knees should hang just past the edge of the bench. Without moving your upper body or arching your lower back, slowly draw your heels toward your buttocks as far as you can. At the top of the movement, squeeze your gluteal muscles for 2 seconds, then slowly lower your legs back down until they are straight once again, and repeat.

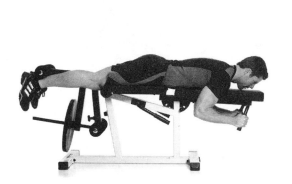 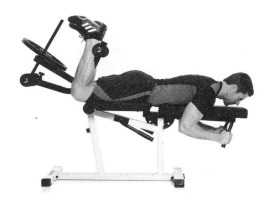

Got additional equipment?

Lie on your back on the floor and place your calves up on a stability ball. Your arms should be at your sides—palms flat on the floor—for balance. Raise your butt off the floor by pushing your hips upward until your body forms a straight line from your shoulders to your knees. Pull your heels toward you and roll the ball as close as possible to your butt. Pause, and reverse the motion—rolling the ball back until your body is straight once again, then lowering your butt back to the floor, and repeat.

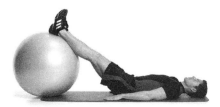 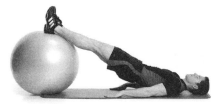 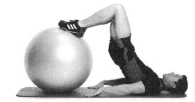

Got nothing to use?

Stand in front of a pair of dumbbells with your feet hip width apart and your knees unlocked. Bending only at your waist, reach down and grab the dumbbells so that your palms face in toward your feet. Keeping your back flat and your legs straight (knees unlocked), slowly raise yourself back up into a standing position until the weights end up in front of your thighs. Resist the urge to pull with your arms; they should stay straight throughout the exercise. Pause, lower the weights back to the floor, and repeat.

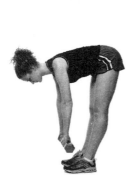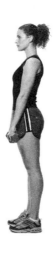

Anytime Exercise #21: LEG EXTENSION

WHAT'S IT WORKING? Your quadriceps

Get it right for more results!

Sit on an exercise bench with a leg-extension attachment, and place your ankles under the footpads. Your back and butt should be flush against the seat. Slowly extend your legs up and forward until they are both straight in front of you, knees unlocked. Pause, slowly bend your knees to lower your legs back down, and repeat.

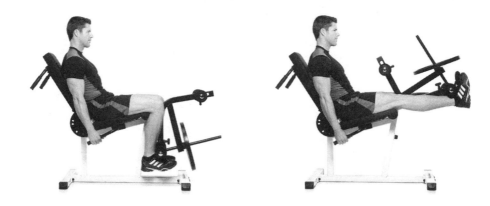

Got additional equipment?

For this variation, you'll strengthen your muscles not by raising the weight but by resisting against it throughout the entire exercise, so grab a partner to help you. Sit at a leg-extension machine and tuck your ankles under the pads. With your back and butt flat against the seat, slowly extend your legs up and forward—having a partner lift the entire bulk of the weight for you with the move—until your legs are extended straight out in front of you, knees unlocked. Keeping your left leg straight, lower your right foot back down so that only your left leg is supporting the weight. (Don't worry! Your muscles can support almost twice as much weight in the lowering phase of an exercise as in the lifting phase.) Pause, then slowly bend your left leg and lower your left foot. Straighten both legs again—letting your partner do all the work—until they are both extended in front of you. This time, keep your right leg straight as you lower your left foot. Pause, then slowly lower your right foot—that's 1 repetition. Continue alternating from left to right throughout the exercise.

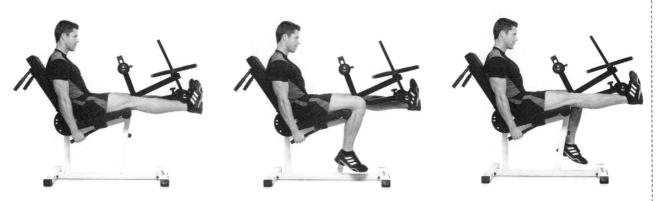

Got nothing to use?

Stand with your back to a sturdy chair, holding a pair of dumbbells with your arms down at your sides and your palms facing in. Rest the top of your right foot on the seat behind you. (Your right leg should be suspended off the ground.) Slowly bend your left leg until you've lowered yourself about 6 to 8 inches (about one-quarter of the way down). Raise yourself back up, and repeat. After you've completed the set on your left side, switch positions to work your right leg.

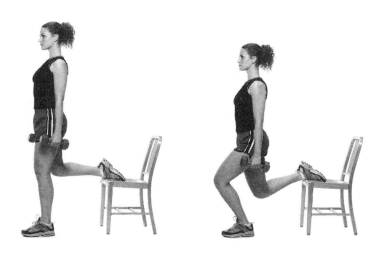

Anytime Exercise #22: LUNGE

WHAT'S IT WORKING? Your quadriceps and gluteal muscles

Get it right for more results!

Stand with your feet hip width apart and rest a light barbell comfortably across your shoulders. Step forward as far as you can with your right foot, bending your right knee so that it's directly above your ankle. (Your right thigh should be parallel to the floor.) Your left leg should stay behind you, with just the ball of your left foot still on the floor. Step back into a standing position, then step out once more, this time with your left leg. That's 1 repetition.

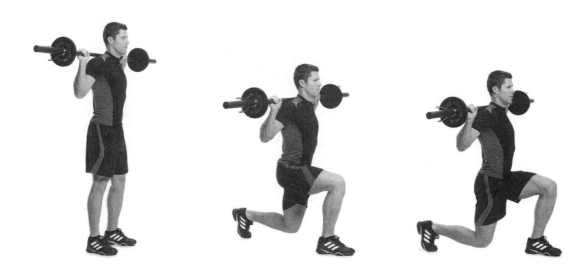

Got additional equipment?

With your right hand, grab the handle of a low cable pulley and stand facing the weight stack, palm facing to the left. Step back so that you're 3 to 4 feet away from the weight stack, with your right arm extended at a low angle in front of you. Keeping your back straight, step forward as far as you can with your left foot until your left thigh is parallel to the floor. Step back into a standing position, and repeat. After your set, switch positions—grabbing the handle with your left hand and stepping forward with your right foot—to work your right leg.

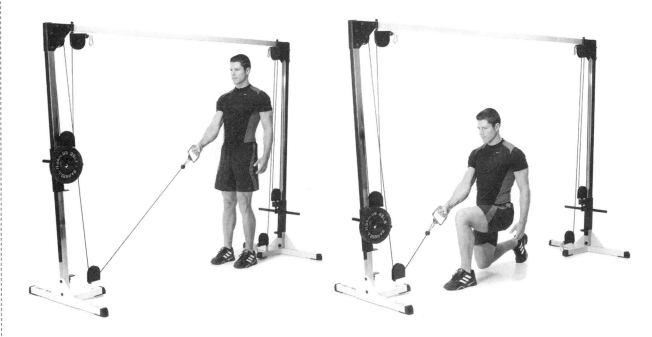

Got nothing to use?

Stand with a dumbbell in each hand, palms facing in, your arms hanging at your sides, and your feet about hip width apart. Keeping your back straight, step forward with your right foot and lean forward until your right thigh is almost parallel to the floor. Gently push yourself back into the starting position, and repeat, this time stepping out with your left foot. That's 1 repetition.

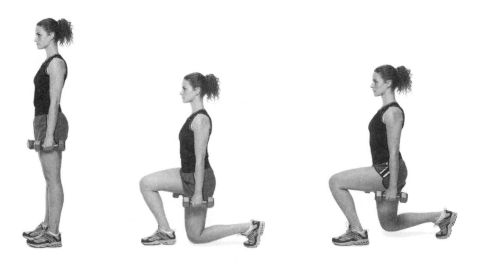

Anytime Exercise #23: LYING TRICEPS PRESS

WHAT'S IT WORKING? Your triceps

Get it right for more results!

Lie flat on a bench, holding a light barbell with a narrow grip—hands no more than 6 inches apart—with your palms facing toward your feet. Press the bar up to arm's length directly above your shoulders. Keeping your shoulders and upper arms stationary, bend your elbows and slowly lower the bar in a semicircular motion down to your forehead. Reverse the motion so that the bar is once again overhead, and repeat.

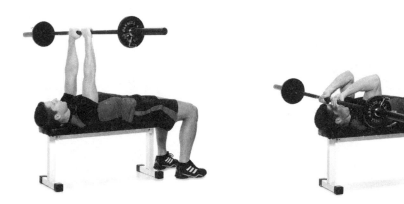

Got additional equipment?

Lie on a decline bench with your head and back resting flat against it. Have a partner hand you an E-Z curl bar, and grab it with your hands about 6 inches apart. Press the bar straight up so that the bar is directly over your head, your palms facing toward your feet. Bending your elbows, lower the weight in a semicircular motion until the bar reaches your forehead. Press the weight back up until it's straight above your head again, and repeat.

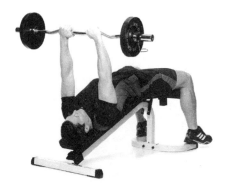
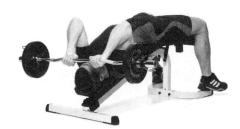

Got nothing to use?

Lie flat on the floor with your knees bent and hold a light dumbbell in each hand. Extend your arms straight up above your shoulders, your palms facing your feet. Keeping your upper arms stationary, slowly bend your elbows and lower the weights down to the sides of your head. Simultaneously rotate your wrists outward as you go, so that your palms face in toward your ears at the bottom of the movement. Press the weights back above you, twisting the weights inward so your palms end up facing your feet, and repeat.

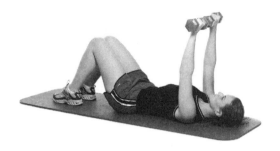 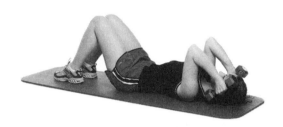

Anytime Exercise #24: ONE-ARM ROW

WHAT'S IT WORKING? Your middle back, latissimus dorsi, rhomboids, trapezius, biceps, and brachioradialis

Get it right for more results!

Stand with your left side to an exercise bench and a dumbbell in your right hand. Rest your left hand and knee on the bench, bend at the waist, and let your right arm hang down toward the floor, your palm facing in toward the bench. Slowly draw the weight up close to your body until it reaches your chest. Lower it until your right arm is straight again, and repeat. After the set, switch sides and hold the weight in your left hand to work your left arm.

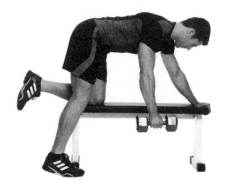 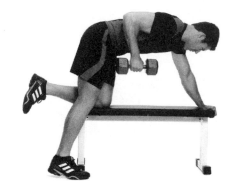

Got additional equipment?

Sit on the edge of an exercise bench facing a low cable pulley. Lean forward and grab the handle with your left hand, then lean back until you are sitting erect, with your left arm fully extended in front of you. With your palm facing down, slowly bring your elbow back as far as possible, keeping it close to your side. Twist your wrist as you go so your thumb ends up pointing toward the ceiling. Slowly return the weight to the starting position, rotating your wrist so your palm ends up facing down, and repeat. Once you've finished the set, switch arms to work your right side.

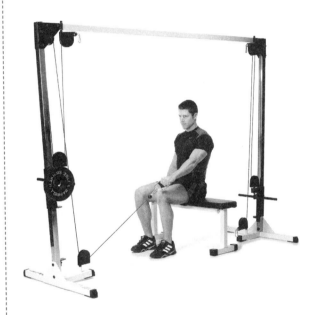 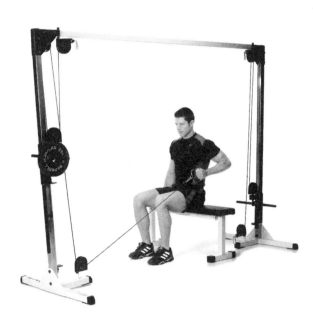

Anytime Exercise #25: ONE-ARM TRICEPS EXTENSION

WHAT'S IT WORKING? Your triceps

Get it right for more results!

Sit on the edge of an exercise bench with a light dumbbell in your right hand. Raise the weight straight up over your head and rotate the dumbbell so that your right palm faces left. Press your right biceps against the side of your head, using your left hand to support your right elbow. Slowly lower the weight behind your head as far as you can, keeping your wrist straight throughout the exercise. Raise the weight overhead until your arm is straight. Repeat for 1 set, then switch hands to work your left arm.

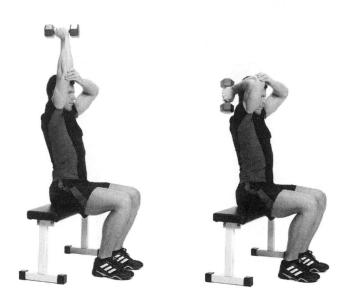

Got additional equipment?

Sit on the edge of an exercise bench about 2 feet away from a high cable pulley. Your knees should be slightly wider than shoulder width apart and your feet should be flat on the floor. Grasp the pulley with your right hand, palm up, and rest your upper right arm against your inner right knee. Rest your left hand on your left knee for support. Slowly extend your right arm, pulling the cable down toward your ankle until your arm is straight. Pause, slowly return to the starting position. Repeat for 1 set, then switch positions to work your left arm.

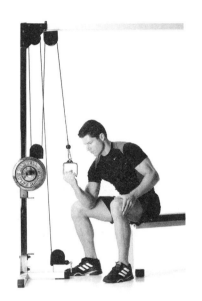 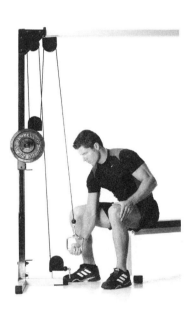

Anytime Exercise #26: POWER CLEAN

WHAT'S IT WORKING? Your thighs, hips, lower back, abdominals, trapezius, shoulders, biceps, and forearms

Get it right for more results!

Stand with your feet shoulder width apart in front of a light barbell and squat down, grabbing the bar with an overhand grip, just outside your feet. Your shoulders should be directly above the bar, legs bent at a 90-degree angle. This is the start of the exercise. Keeping your back straight and your head facing forward, quickly stand up and pull the weight off the floor, letting the bar rise up close to your body. As you quickly shrug the weight up to chest height, rise up on your toes. Immediately bend your knees slightly to get below the weight, and rotate your arms underneath the bar to catch it—the bar should come to rest across the front of your shoulders. Pause, then reverse the motion to return the bar to the floor, and repeat.

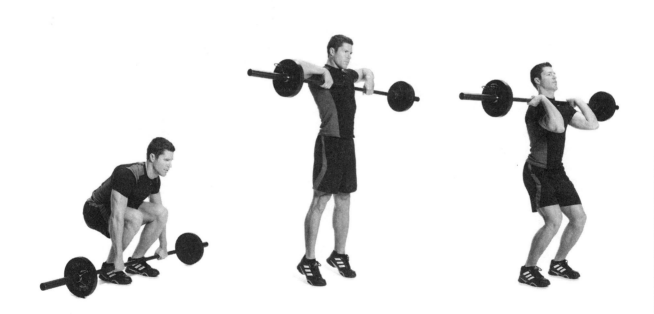

Got nothing to use?

Stand with your feet shoulder width apart and place a dumbbell in front of each foot. Bend your knees and grab the dumbbells with your palms facing toward you. This is the start of the exercise. Keeping your back straight and your head facing forward, quickly stand up and pull the weights off the floor, letting the dumbbells rise up close to your body. As you quickly shrug the weights up to chest height, rise up on your toes. Immediately bend your knees slightly to get below the weights, and rotate your arms underneath the weights to catch them—the weights should end up resting across the front of your shoulders. Pause, then reverse the motion to return the weights to the floor, and repeat.

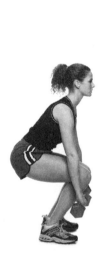 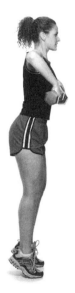 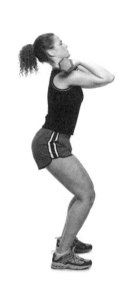

Anytime Exercise #27: PREACHER CURL

WHAT'S IT WORKING? Your biceps

Get it right for more results!

Sit at a preacher-curl station holding a light barbell in both hands, your palms facing up. Rest your upper arms on the slanted pad in front of you. Keeping your back straight, slowly curl the barbell up until it reaches your shoulders. Slowly lower the weight back down, and repeat.

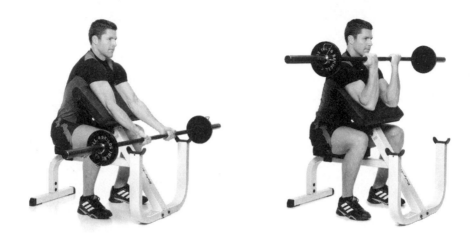

Got additional equipment?

Grab an E-Z curl bar with an underhand grip, and kneel behind a stability ball. Keeping your upper arms planted on the ball, curl the weight up as high as you can. Resist the urge to lean back—you want your biceps to do all the work. Pause, slowly lower the bar back down, and repeat.

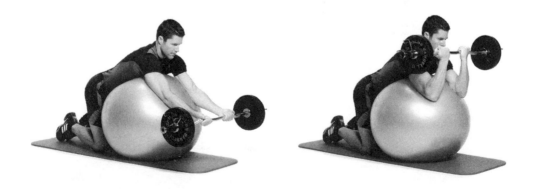

Got nothing to use?

Sit on the edge of a chair with a light dumbbell in your right hand. Keeping your back straight, bend at the waist so that your right arm hangs down between your legs. The back of your right arm should rest on the inside of your right thigh, palm facing in. (Your left hand can rest on your left knee.) Keeping your upper arm pressed against your thigh, slowly curl the weight up to your right shoulder. Lower the weight back down until your arm hangs straight once again, and repeat. Afterward, switch positions to work your left arm.

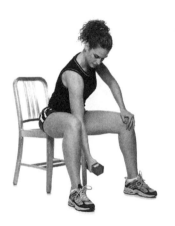 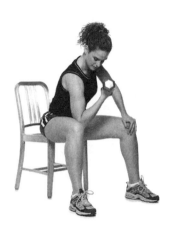

Anytime Exercise #28: PULLOVER

WHAT'S IT WORKING? Your upper back, lower pectorals, and triceps

Get it right for more results!

Lie flat on an exercise bench with your feet flat on the floor. Grab a light dumbbell and hold it vertically over your chest with both hands, wrapping your thumbs and fingers close around the handle so that the bottom of the top part of the dumbbell rests flat on your hands. Your palms should face up toward the ceiling. Keeping your elbows slightly bent, slowly lower the weight backward in an arc over your head until you feel a slight stretch in your sides and your upper arms are in line with your head. Slowly pull the weight back up until it's once again overhead, and repeat.

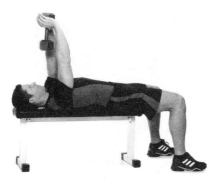 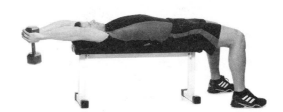

Got additional equipment?

Hook a two-handed rope handle to a low pulley, then position an exercise bench lengthwise about 2 feet from it. Lie down on the bench—with your head on the end toward the pulley—and reach back and grab the rope with both hands. Your arms should be extended behind you—palms facing each other—with your upper arms positioned alongside your ears. Keeping your arms slightly bent, slowly pull your arms up and forward until your hands are straight up above your chest. Pause, slowly resist the weight as you reverse the motion, and repeat.

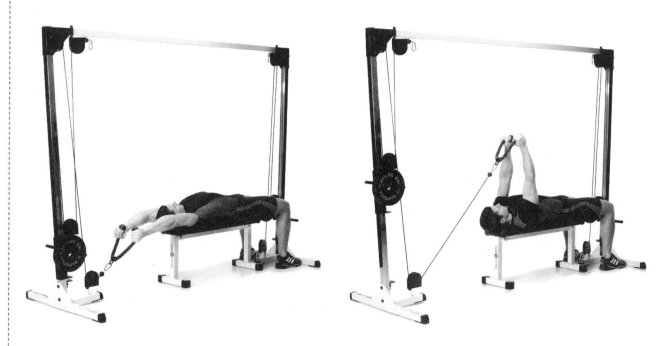

Anytime Exercise #29: PUSH PRESS

WHAT'S IT WORKING? Your thighs, chest, shoulders, and triceps

Get it right for more results!

Stand with a light barbell across the front of your shoulders, your hands slightly wider than shoulder width apart, palms facing forward and elbows pointing down. Raise your forearms until they are almost parallel to the ground. (Your elbows should be pointing ahead of you.) Squat down about 6 inches, look up, then quickly rise back up, pushing off the balls of your feet. As you begin to ascend, shrug your shoulders up so the bar lifts off your chest (this spares your wrists from straining to raise off the bar), then press the weight up over your head until the bar is directly overhead, elbows locked. Lower the weight back down to your shoulders, and repeat.

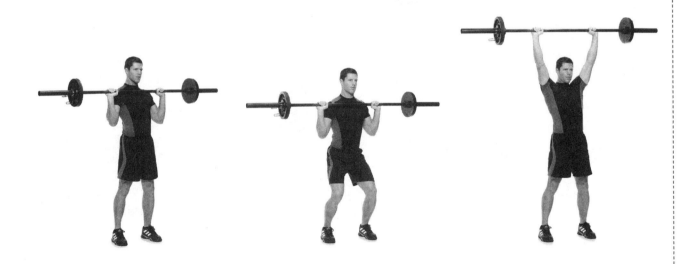

Got nothing to use?

Stand holding a light dumbbell in each hand in front of your shoulders. Your arms should be bent—elbows pointing down—with your palms facing forward. Raise your forearms until they are almost parallel to the ground. (Your elbows should be pointing ahead of you.) Squat down about 6 inches, look up, then quickly rise back up, pushing off the balls of your feet. As you begin to ascend, shrug your shoulders up so the weights lift off your chest, then press them up over your head. Lower the weights back down to your shoulders, and repeat.

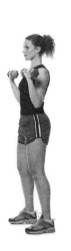
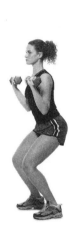
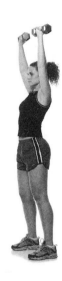

Anytime Exercise #30: REVERSE CRUNCH

WHAT'S IT WORKING? Your lower rectus abdominis

Get it right for more results!

Get on the floor as if you were about to perform a pushup—placing your hands shoulder width apart. But instead of straightening your legs with your feet on the floor, rest the front of your shins on a stability ball. With your arms straight and your back flat, your body should form a straight line from your shoulders to your ankles. Slowly roll the ball forward with your feet, toward your chest, raising your hips and rounding your back as you go. Pause, return to the starting position, and repeat.

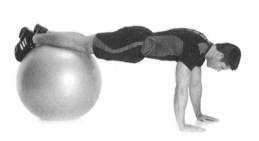 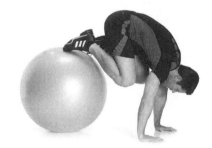

Got additional equipment?

Hang from a chinup bar with your arms slightly wider than shoulder width apart, your palms facing forward, and your legs straight. (If you're tall, you may need to start with your knees bent and your feet behind you.) Keeping your feet together, bend your knees and slowly raise them to your chest. Pause for 2 seconds, then slowly lower them back down until your legs are straight again, and repeat.

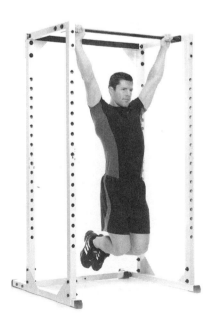 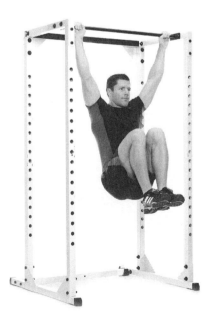

Got nothing to use?

Lie flat on your back with your arms straight at your sides, palms flat on the floor. Keeping your legs together, bend your knees and draw them up until your legs form a 90-degree angle. (Your thighs should be perpendicular to the floor.) Slowly lift your butt off the floor and curl your pelvis toward your rib cage. Your knees should automatically curl toward your chest. Pause, then slowly lower your butt back down to the floor, and repeat.

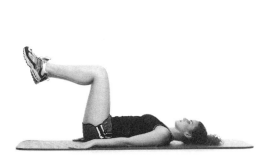 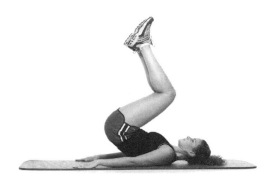

Anytime Exercise #31: REVERSE CURL

WHAT'S IT WORKING? Your biceps and forearms

Get it right for more results!

Grab a barbell with an overhand grip and your hands shoulder width apart. Your arms should hang straight so that the bar rests right in front of your legs, your palms facing in toward your thighs. Keeping your back straight and your elbows tucked into your sides, slowly curl the bar up in a semicircular motion until the tops of your forearms touch your biceps. Pause, slowly lower the bar back down in front of your legs, and repeat.

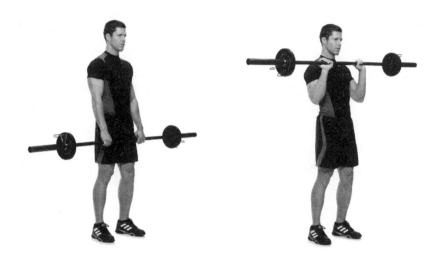

Got additional equipment?

Attach a straight bar to a low cable pulley and stand facing the weight stack, about 1 to 2 feet away. Grab the bar with an overhand grip—palms facing down—with your hands about shoulder width apart. With your elbows fixed at your sides, slowly curl the bar up until it's just below your chin. Pause, lower the bar back down in front of you, and repeat.

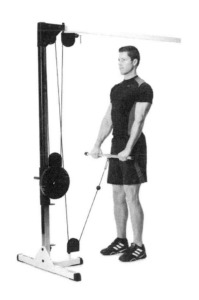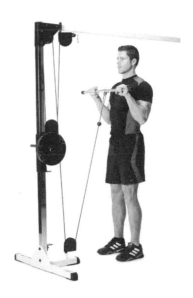

Got nothing to use?

Stand straight with a dumbbell in each hand, your arms down in front of you. Your palms should be facing the fronts of your thighs. Keeping your back straight, slowly curl both dumbbells toward your shoulders, keeping your wrists from turning as you go. The backs of your hands should be facing the front of your shoulders at the top of the move. Slowly lower the weights back down until your arms are straight, and repeat.

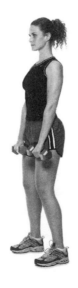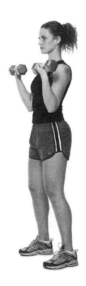

Anytime Exercise #32: REVERSE LUNGE

WHAT'S IT WORKING? Your quadriceps, hamstrings, gluteal muscles, and calves

Get it right for more results!

Stand with your feet hip width apart, a light barbell resting comfortably across your shoulders. Keeping your back straight, step backward with your left foot and lower your hips until your right thigh is parallel to the floor. Slowly push yourself back up into a standing position, and repeat, this time stepping back with your right foot. That's 1 repetition. Continue alternating from left to right throughout the exercise.

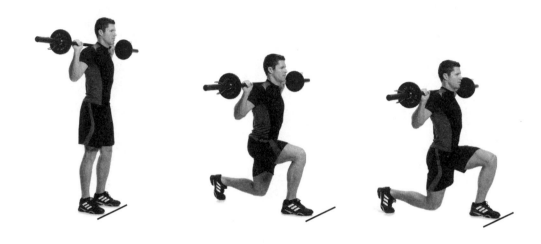

Got additional equipment?

With your right hand, grab the handle of a low cable pulley and stand facing the weight stack, palm facing to the left. You should be far enough away so that your right arm is extended at a low angle in front of you. Keeping your back straight, step backward with your right foot and lower your hips until your left thigh is parallel to the floor. Slowly push yourself back up, and repeat. Complete your repetitions on that side, then switch positions—grabbing the handle with your left hand and stepping back with your left foot—to work your left leg.

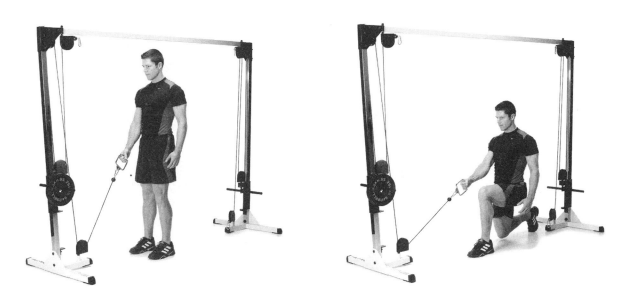

Got nothing to use?

Stand with a dumbbell in each hand, palms facing in, your arms hanging at your sides, and your feet shoulder width apart. Keeping your back straight, step backward with your left foot and lower your hips until your right thigh is parallel to the floor. Slowly push yourself back up, and repeat, this time stepping back with your right foot. That's 1 repetition. Continue alternating from left to right throughout the exercise.

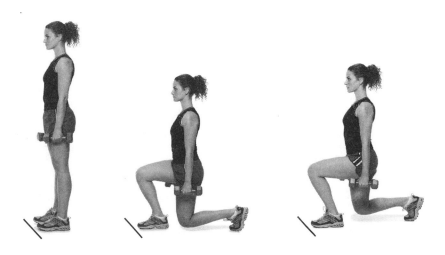

Anytime Exercise #33: SEATED CALF RAISE

WHAT'S IT WORKING? Your calf muscles

Get it right for more results!

Place a step or a block of wood in front of a bench, then grab a pair of dumbbells and sit down on the bench. Set the balls of both feet on the step, and place one weight vertically on each knee. Push up on the toes of your feet to raise your heels as high as you can. Pause, lower your heels down to the floor as far as you can, and repeat.

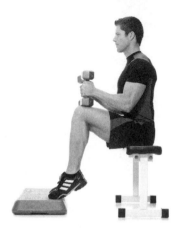 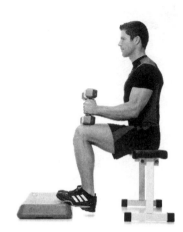

Got additional equipment?

Sit at a seated calf machine with your knees under the pads and your feet on the step, your heels hanging off the edge. Slowly lift up on the balls of your feet as high as you can. Pause, slowly lower your heels as far as possible to the floor, and repeat.

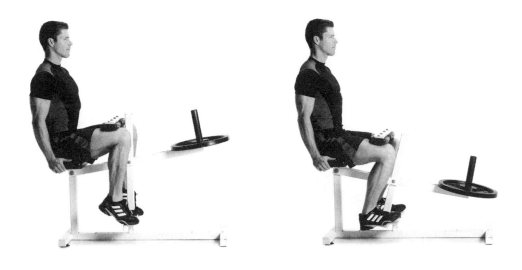

Anytime Exercise #34: SEATED SHOULDER PRESS

WHAT'S IT WORKING? Your anterior and medial deltoids and triceps

Get it right for more results!

Sit on the end of an exercise bench, with your feet flat on the floor and a barbell lying over the tops of your thighs. Grab the barbell in an overhand grip, with your hands slightly wider than shoulder width apart, and raise it so that the middle of the bar rests directly above the top of your chest. Keeping your back straight and your head facing forward, slowly press the bar over your head until your arms are straight, elbows unlocked. Lower the bar back down to your chest, and repeat.

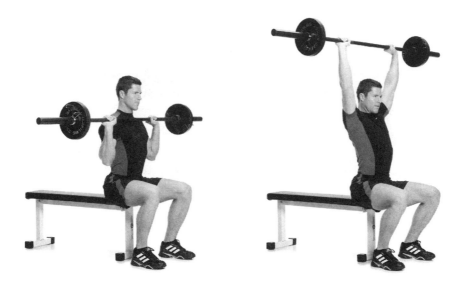

Got additional equipment?

Sit down on a stability ball with a dumbbell in each hand. To help maintain your balance, spread your feet slightly wider than shoulder width apart, keeping your feet flat on the floor. Bring the weights up to the sides of your shoulders, your palms facing forward. Keeping your back straight, slowly press the weights over your head until your arms are straight, elbows unlocked. Lower the weights back down to your shoulders, and repeat.

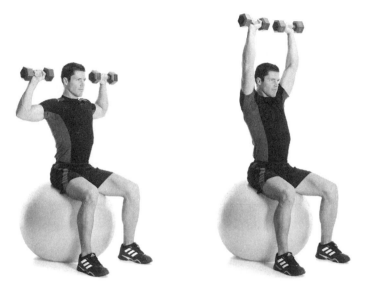

Got nothing to use?

Sit on a chair with your feet firmly on the floor and a dumbbell in each hand. Bring the weights to the sides of your shoulders, your palms facing forward. Slowly press the weights over your head, keeping your back straight as you go. Lower them back down to your shoulders, and repeat.

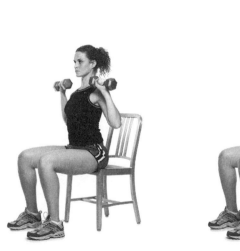
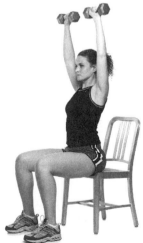

Anytime Exercise #35: SEATED TRICEPS EXTENSION

WHAT'S IT WORKING? Your triceps

Get it right for more results!

Sit on a bench with your back straight, place your feet firmly on the floor, and grasp a single dumbbell with both hands. Raise the weight above your head, rotating it so that it's vertical and the top plate rests comfortably on the palms of your hands. Your thumbs should be wrapped around the handle for safety. Slowly lower the weight behind your head until your forearms touch your biceps. Press the weight back over your head, and repeat.

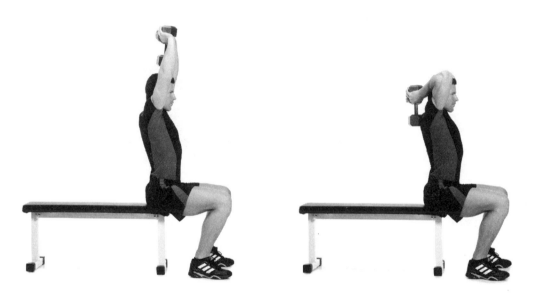

Got additional equipment?

Attach a V-shaped bar to a low cable pulley system and kneel with your back to the weight stack. (If you don't have a V-bar, use an attachable rope or thread a small, thick towel through the end of the cable instead.) Grab both handles and straighten your arms overhead, your palms facing forward (the bottom of the V should be pointing down). Keeping your upper arms stationary, slowly bend your elbows and lower your hands behind your neck. Reverse the motion by straightening your arms back over your head, and repeat.

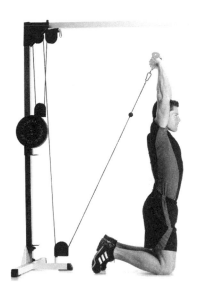 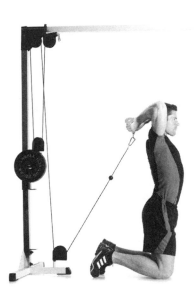

Anytime Exercise #36: SHRUG

WHAT'S IT WORKING? Your trapezius and forearms

Get it right for more results!

Grab a barbell with an overhand grip—your palms facing toward you, and your hands shoulder width apart. Your arms should hang straight so that the bar touches the fronts of your thighs. Keeping your back straight, slowly raise your shoulders as high as you can. Pause, slowly lower your shoulders until your arms hang down as far as possible, and repeat.

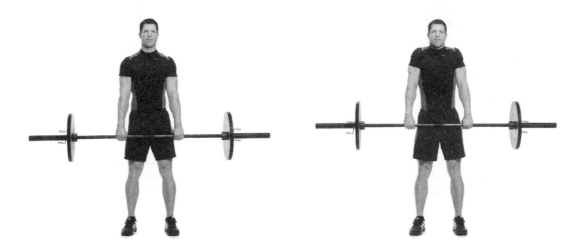

Got additional equipment?

Attach a straight bar to a low cable pulley and stand facing the weight stack, about 1 to 2 feet away. Grab the bar with an overhand grip—palms facing toward your thighs—with your hands shoulder width apart. Slowly raise your shoulders as high as you can. Pause, then lower them, and repeat.

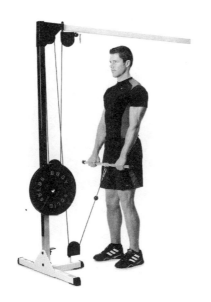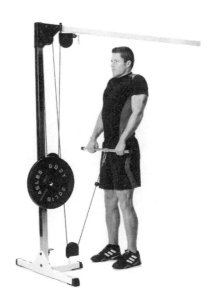

Got nothing to use?

Sit on a chair with a dumbbell in each hand. Your arms should be hanging at your sides, with your palms facing each other. With your back straight and your head facing forward, slowly raise your shoulders as high as you can. Pause, slowly lower your shoulders, and repeat.

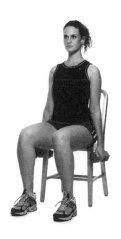 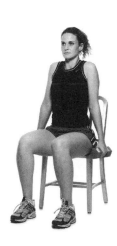

Anytime Exercise #37: SIDE LUNGE

WHAT'S IT WORKING? Your quadriceps, hamstrings, gluteal muscles, and calves

Get it right for more results!

Stand straight with your feet shoulder width apart and a dumbbell in each hand, your arms down at your sides, palms facing each other. Step out with your right foot, placing it slightly forward and a couple of feet to the right. Lean onto your right leg until your right thigh is almost parallel to the floor, then push yourself back into a standing position. Repeat the move on the left side using your left leg, lowering yourself down until your left thigh is almost parallel to the floor. That's 1 repetition. Continue lunging from right to left throughout the exercise.

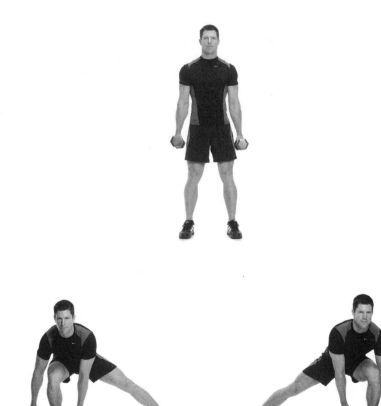

Got additional equipment?

Place a light barbell on a squat rack and stand in front of it. Step forward, grab the bar with an overhand grip slightly wider than shoulder width apart, and rest the bar across the back of your shoulders. Step back and space your feet slightly wider than shoulder width apart. Slowly begin to bend just your right knee, keeping your back flat and the bar steady as you go, until your right thigh is almost parallel to the floor. Slowly push yourself back up until your knees are almost in a locked position. Repeat the move to the left side, lowering yourself down until your left thigh is almost parallel to the floor. That's 1 repetition. Continue lunging from right to left throughout the exercise.

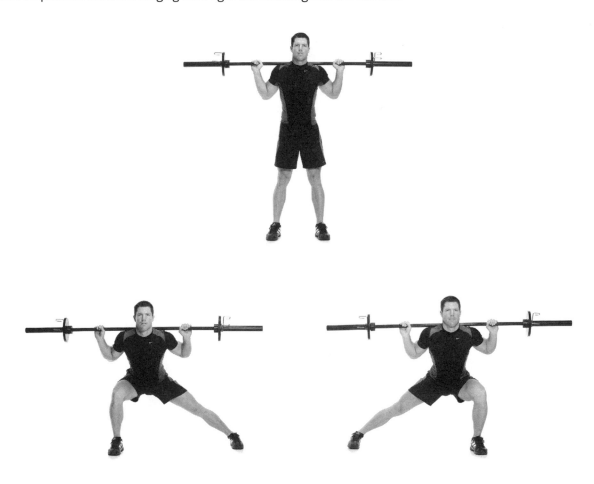

Anytime Exercise #38: SIDE RAISE

WHAT'S IT WORKING? Your obliques

Get it right for more results!

Lie flat on the floor with your knees bent, your feet together, and your hands resting lightly along the sides of your ears. Keeping your legs and feet together, twist at the waist and lean your legs over to your right. Curl your torso up and forward, raising your shoulders off the floor. Pause, lower yourself, and repeat. Finish the set, then switch sides—leaning your legs over to the left—and repeat the exercise.

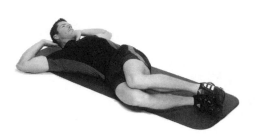 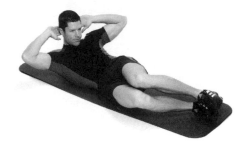

Got additional equipment?

Get on your knees with your right side toward the weight stack of a high cable pulley. Grab the handle with your right hand and pull it down by the right side of your head, your palm facing in. Keeping the handle by your head, curl your rib cage to the right toward your pelvis. Rise up and repeat. After your set, switch positions—your left side should now be toward the weight stack—and repeat the exercise.

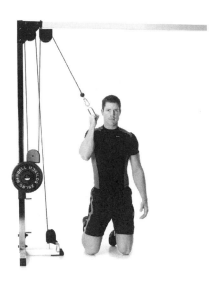 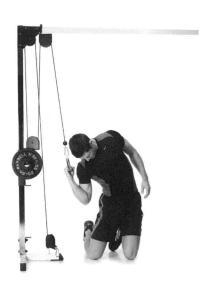

Anytime Exercise #39: SQUAT

WHAT'S IT WORKING? Your quadriceps, hamstrings, gluteal muscles, and calves

Get it right for more results!

Place a barbell on a squat rack and stand in front of it. Grab the bar with an overhand grip slightly wider than shoulder width apart, duck underneath it, and rest the bar across the back of your shoulders. With your feet hip width apart and your back straight, slowly squat down until your thighs are almost parallel to the floor. Slowly push yourself back up, and repeat.

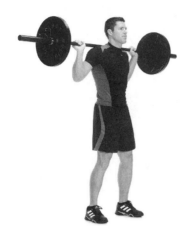 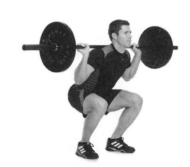

Got additional equipment?

Sit in a leg-press machine with your feet shoulder width apart against the platform. Grip the handles at your sides for support as you bend your knees, stopping when your legs form a 90-degree angle. (Any farther could put too much stress on your knee joints.) Press the weight back up until your legs are straight with your knees unlocked, and repeat.

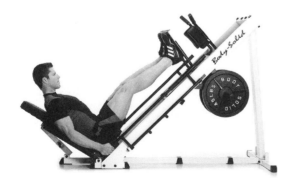 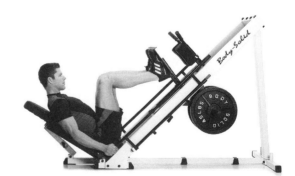

Got nothing to use?

Stand 18 to 24 inches away from a sturdy wall, facing away from it. Lean back so that your head, shoulders, back, and butt rest flat against the wall. Lift your right foot and tuck it behind your left calf. Slowly bend your left leg and lower yourself down, sliding along the wall, until your left thigh is almost parallel to the floor. Pause, then push yourself back up into a standing position. Do all your repetitions on that side, then switch leg positions to work your right leg.

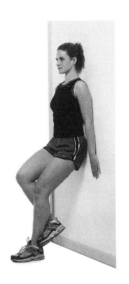 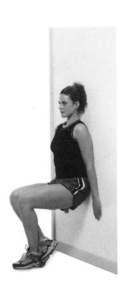

Anytime Exercise #40: STANDING CALF RAISE

WHAT'S IT WORKING? Your calf muscles

Get it right for more results!

Grab a dumbbell in your right hand, palm facing in, and stand on the second step of a staircase. The balls of your feet should rest on the edge of the step so that your heels hang off the edge. Place your left hand against a wall for support, and tuck your left foot behind your right ankle. Slowly rise up on the toes of your right foot, raising your right heel up as high as you can. Pause, then slowly lower your right heel down as far as possible. Once you have finished your set, switch positions to work your left leg.

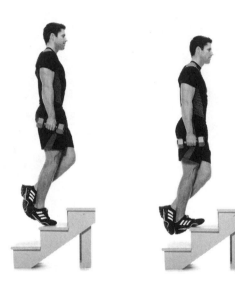

Got additional equipment?

Sit in a leg-press machine with your legs straight and your feet close together. Instead of placing your feet flat on the platform, slide them down so that just the balls of your feet are resting on it—your heels should rest just below the platform. Keeping your legs straight, slowly push the platform up with just the balls of your feet. Slowly return the platform to the starting position, and repeat.

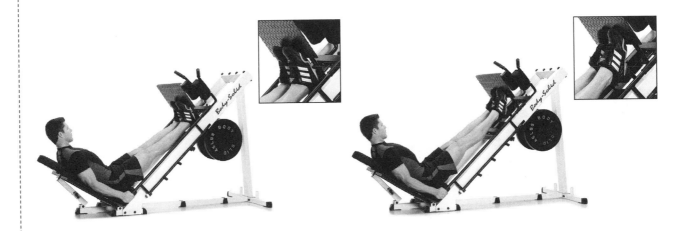

Anytime Exercise #41: TRICEPS PUSHDOWN

WHAT'S IT WORKING? Your triceps

Get it right for more results!

Stand in front of a high pulley station and grab the bar with an overhand grip, your hands 6 inches apart. Keeping your back straight, tuck your upper arms into your sides and position your forearms so that they're parallel to the floor. Your elbows should be pointing straight behind you. Slowly push the bar down until your arms are straight and the bar reaches the fronts of your thighs. Pause, slowly raise the bar back up until your forearms are parallel to the floor, and repeat.

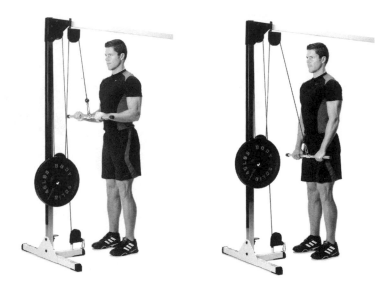

Got additional equipment?

This variation can be done without a partner, but it's much safer for your lower back to have someone assist you.

Lie faceup on an exercise bench with your knees bent and your feet flat on the floor. Have your partner hand you a barbell, and grab it with an overhand grip, your hands less than shoulder width apart. Raise the bar so that your arms are fully extended above your chest, with your elbows unlocked and your palms facing toward your feet. Slowly lower the bar down and back until it reaches your head, then press the weight back overhead, elbows unlocked, and repeat.

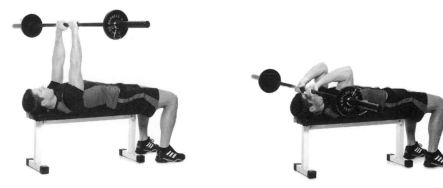

Got nothing to use?

Sit on a sturdy chair and shuffle your butt forward, placing your palms on the chair with your fingers hanging off the front edge. Keeping your hands in place, slowly step forward until your legs are in front of you. Your arms should be straight with elbows unlocked, supporting your weight behind you. Slowly lower yourself until your butt is as close to the floor as possible without touching it. Press back up until your arms are straight, elbows unlocked, and repeat.

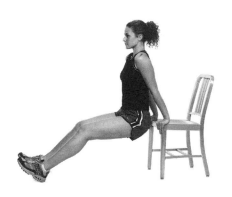 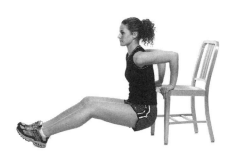

Anytime Exercise #42: TWISTING CRUNCH

WHAT'S IT WORKING? Your upper rectus abdominis

Get it right for more results!

Sit on top of a stability ball with your legs in front of you and your feet flat on the floor. Cross your arms across your chest, touching each hand to the opposite shoulder (left hand on your right shoulder, and vice versa). Keeping your feet flat on the floor, slowly lean back and roll yourself down the ball until your head, shoulders, and back touch it. Slowly curl your head, arms, and upper back off the ball and twist your torso to the right. Lower back down onto the ball and repeat the move, this time twisting yourself to the left. That's 1 repetition.

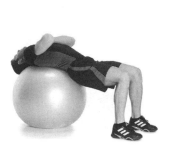 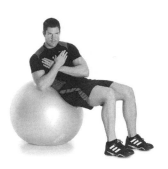 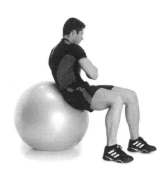

Got additional equipment?

Get on your knees in front of a high cable pulley with a rope attachment, and grab both ends of the rope. Pulling it over the back of your neck, draw your hands either down by the sides of your ears (palms facing in) or just down below your chin (palms touching the top of your chest). Keeping your hands locked in place, slowly curl yourself down and forward, starting by drawing your chin toward your chest, then letting your shoulders and back follow. Curl yourself down and to the left as far as you comfortably can, then slowly reverse the motion to come back up. Repeat the exercise, this time curling yourself down and to the right. That's 1 repetition.

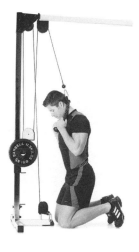 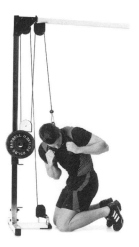 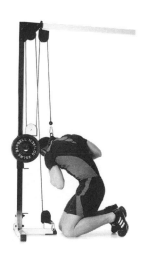

Got nothing to use?

Lie on your back with your legs bent and your feet flat on the floor. Touch your hands lightly to the sides of your head with your elbows pointing out to the sides. Slowly lift your shoulders off the ground and twist your body to the left so that your right elbow points toward your knees. Lower yourself back down and repeat the movement, this time twisting to the right so that your left elbow points toward your knees. That's 1 repetition.

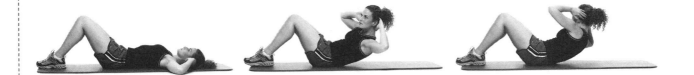

Anytime Exercise #43: TWISTING LEG THRUST

WHAT'S IT WORKING? Your lower rectus abdominis and obliques

Get it right for more results!

Lie on your back with your knees bent and your feet flat on the floor. Tuck your hands underneath your pelvis, palms down, along the sides of your tailbone. Keeping your knees in a bent position, slowly raise your feet about 18 inches. This is the starting position. Begin to extend your legs straight into the air as high as you can. At the top of the movement, twist your hips to the left (your feet should point to the left). Lower your legs back down into the starting position (your feet suspended off the floor) and repeat the move, this time twisting your hips to the right. That's 1 repetition.

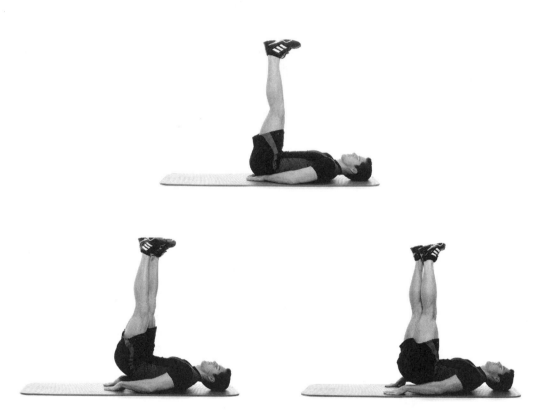

Got additional equipment?

Have a partner tuck a small medicine ball (1 to 2 pounds, to start) between your feet and squeeze it in place as you perform the same exercise. The added weight will create even greater resistance on your abdominal muscles.

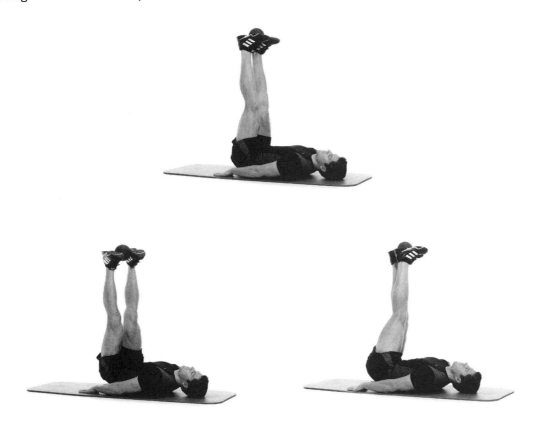

Anytime Exercise #44: TWISTING TOE TOUCH

WHAT'S IT WORKING? Your upper and lower rectus abdominis and obliques

Get it right for more results!

Lie flat on your back, and raise your arms and legs straight up so that your hands and feet point to the ceiling. Holding this position, slowly curl up, twist to the left, and touch the outside of your right hand to the outside of your left ankle. Lower and re-peat, this time twisting to the right and touching your left hand to your right ankle. That's 1 repetition.

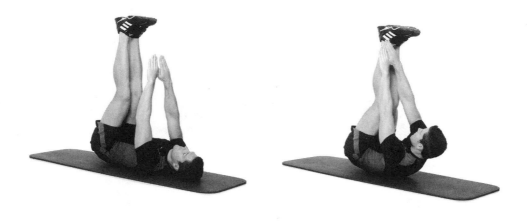

Got additional equipment?

Get into the same position, but grab a light medicine ball with both hands and hold it above you, with your arms extended and your palms facing in toward each other. Holding this position, slowly curl up, twist to the left, and touch your left ankle with the ball. Lower and repeat, this time twisting to the right and touching your right ankle with the ball. That's 1 repetition.

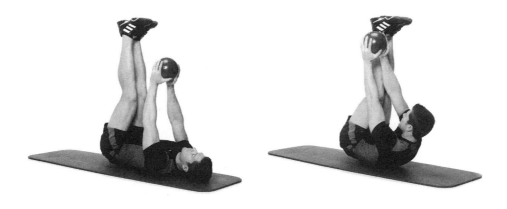

Anytime Exercise #45: UPRIGHT ROW

WHAT'S IT WORKING? Your trapezius and shoulders

Get it right for more results!

Stand straight with your feet shoulder width apart, holding a barbell with your hands spaced 8 to 10 inches apart. Your arms should be hanging straight in front of you, with your palms facing in toward your body. Keeping your back straight, slowly raise the bar straight up, letting your elbows lead the movement, until the bar is directly below your chin. Your elbows should be angled up and pointing to the sides. Slowly lower the bar back down, and repeat.

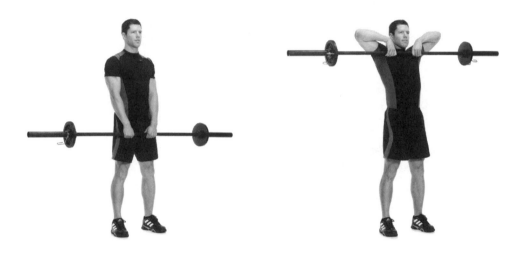

Got additional equipment?

Attach a straight bar to a low cable pulley and stand facing the weight stack, about 1 to 2 feet away. Grab the bar with an overhand grip—your palms facing toward you—with your hands about 6 inches from each other. Keeping your back straight, slowly pull the bar up until it's directly under your chin. Pause, lower the bar back down, and repeat.

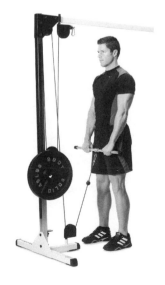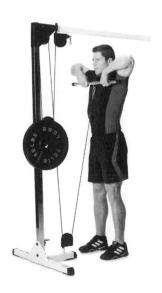

Got nothing to use?

Stand straight, feet shoulder width apart, with a dumbbell in each hand. Let your arms hang straight down in front of you so that the dumbbells rest on your upper thighs, your palms facing your body. Slowly draw the weights up toward your chin. Pause, slowly lower the weights back down, and repeat.

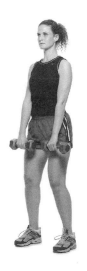 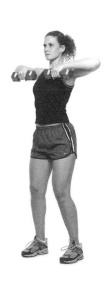

Anytime Exercise #46: V-UP WITH A TWIST

WHAT'S IT WORKING? Your upper and lower rectus abdominis and obliques

Get it right for more results!

Lie flat with your legs straight, your arms at your sides, and your palms facing down. Raise your legs and torso so that they're both at a 45-degree angle. (You should look like the letter V.) Extend your hands as far as you can toward your feet. Hold this starting position, then twist your torso slightly forward and to the left. Rotate back into the starting position, then twist to the right. Lower yourself back to the floor, and repeat.

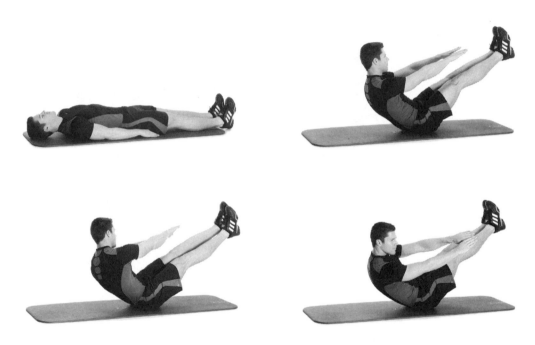

Got additional equipment?

Hold a light medicine ball in your hands, then perform the move as previously instructed. Once you've exhausted your abdominal muscles, drop the medicine ball and finish the set using only your body weight.

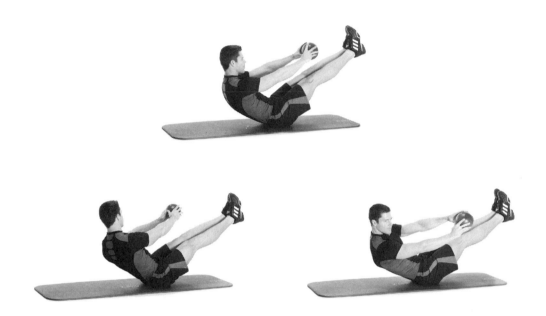

Anytime Exercise #47: WRIST CURL

WHAT'S IT WORKING? Your forearm flexors

Get it right for more results!

Sit on an exercise bench with your knees bent and your feet about shoulder width apart. Grab a very light barbell with both hands in an underhand grip, and place your forearms on your thighs so that the backs of your wrists are extended over your kneecaps. Keeping your forearms flush against your thighs, lower the weight down as far as possible. Curl it back up, and repeat.

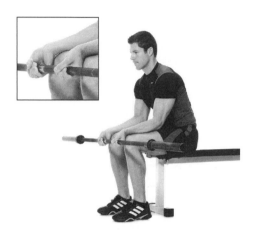 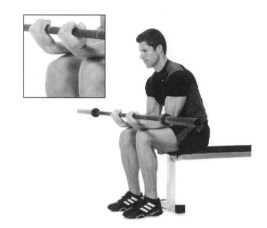

Got additional equipment?

Place an exercise bench perpendicular to a low cable station and attach a two-handed bar to the low pulley. Kneel on the opposite side of the bench and grab the bar, palms up, placing your forearms flat on the bench so that only your wrists extend over the edge. Keeping your arms flat, lower your hands down as far as possible. Curl the bar up as far as you can, and repeat.

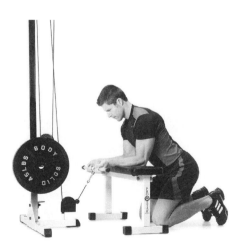 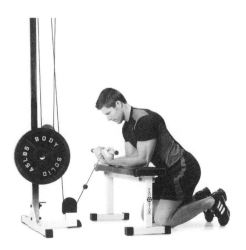

Got nothing to use?

Sit on a chair with your knees bent and your feet about shoulder width apart. Grab a very light dumbbell in each hand and place your forearms on your thighs, palms up, so that the backs of your wrists extend over your kneecaps. Keeping your forearms flush against your thighs, lower the weights down as far as possible. Curl them back up, and repeat.

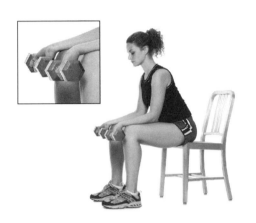 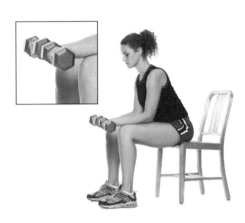

Anytime Exercise #48: WRIST EXTENSION

WHAT'S IT WORKING? Your forearm extensors

Get it right for more results!

Sit on an exercise bench with your knees bent and your feet about shoulder width apart. Grab a very light barbell and place your forearms on your thighs, palms down, so that your wrists extend over your kneecaps. You may have to lean forward slightly to get your forearms flat against your legs. Bending at the wrists, lower the barbell as far as possible while keeping a tight grip. Raise the weight as high as you can, keeping your forearms pressed to the tops of your thighs, and repeat.

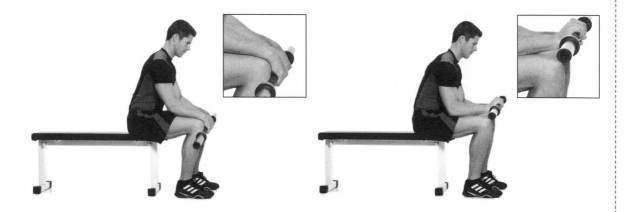

Got additional equipment?

Place an exercise bench perpendicular to a low cable station and attach a two-handed bar to the low pulley. Kneel on the opposite side of the bench and grab the bar, palms down, placing your forearms flat on the bench so that only your wrists extend over the edge. Keeping your arms flat, lower your hands down as far as possible. Curl them back toward you as far as you can, and repeat.

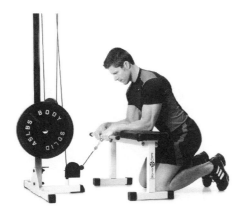
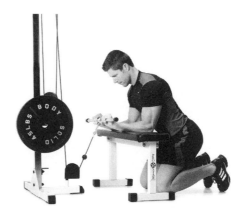

Got nothing to use?

Sit on a chair with your knees bent and your feet about shoulder width apart. Grab a very light dumbbell in each hand and place your forearms on your thighs, palms down, so that your wrists extend over your kneecaps. You may have to lean forward slightly to get your forearms flat against your legs. Bending at the wrists, lower the dumbbells as far as possible while keeping a tight grip. Raise the dumbbells as high as you can, keeping your forearms pressed to the tops of your thighs, and repeat.

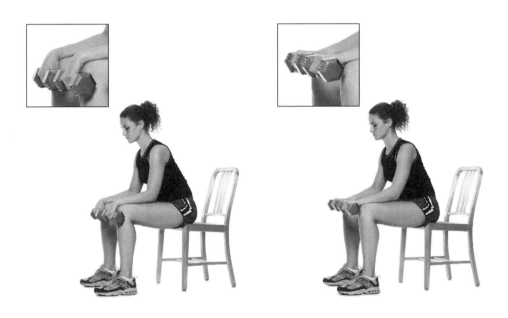

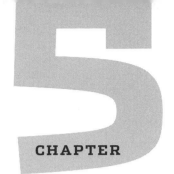

I Have Only 1 Day a Week

Why Just 1 Day Is Still Okay

That's all you have for me, eh?

Don't worry. I'm not here to judge you; I'm here to help.

We've all been in that state of exercise helplessness. Maybe it was a busy workweek spent pleasing your annoying boss or that vacation you took to escape him. Or maybe it was the unexpected foul weather that dropped 24 inches of snow, or your unappreciative mother-in-law who dropped in unexpectedly for a weeklong visit. Whatever the annoyance, whoever the distraction, something has left you with nothing more than 1 day to get the job done.

Most people would pack it in and not bother for the week, but if you're a beginning exerciser looking for results or an expert exerciser looking to keep the results you already have, using that 1 day you *do* have is crucial to keeping you on track.

The truth is, being able to pony up only 1 day a week won't make the same significant changes to your body composition that future workouts—where you have more time to give—will offer. However, it's still a great starting place for ama-

teurs and a great alternative for the experienced exerciser.

Why? Because if a bad week keeps you from exercising as much as you'd like to, research has shown that *all you need to do to maintain your current level of fitness is to exercise just 1 day a week.* That's right. Researchers at Ball State University in Muncie, Indiana, had subjects go through a 12-week strength-training program, then they tested the effectiveness of training just 1 day a week afterward.

Same Time, More Results

USE YOUR BRAIN WHEN YOU'RE NOT USING YOUR BODY.

Getting set up for some exercises can take more than a minute—and that may be time you don't have to spare. Instead of watching the clock between your sets, try thinking ahead to save even more time: See what exercise is coming next, then prepare for it during your breathers by reaching for the weights or setting up the machine you'll need to use. Make the most of those precious seconds, and your muscles will benefit more from the time you *do* have.

Same Time, More Results

KEEP A CLOSE EYE ON WHATEVER BENDS.

Placing the right amount of tension on your muscles is the fastest way to improve your muscles with the least risk of injury. But your knee and elbow joints can interfere with that goal if you don't watch them closely. **Don't be so stiff.** Straightening your arms and legs to the point where your elbow and knee joints lock may give your muscles time to breathe, but it's a snooze that can rob you of results and leave you feeling worse after your workout. In most exercises, locking your joints removes some of the stress of the movement from the muscles you're working and pushes it onto weaker tendons and ligaments within and around your joints. Basically, the tension of the exercise is placed on your bones instead of your muscles.

Don't be so flexible. Overbending your arms or legs can be just as painful. Some exercises—such as lunges, squats, and triceps pushdowns—require that you bend your arms or legs just shy of 90 degrees. Going beyond 90 degrees only redirects stress off of your muscles and forces it onto weaker tendons.

To keep from sabotaging your results, straighten your arms and legs as close to a locking position as possible—but don't lock them. For exercises that require you to bend your arms and legs only to the point of 90 degrees, try doing the exercise with your side turned toward a mirror. That way, you can see whether your arms or legs are bent perfectly: They should resemble the letter L, not a V.

Right

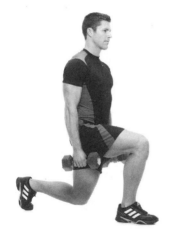

Wrong

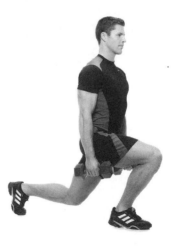

Right

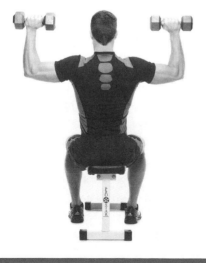

Wrong

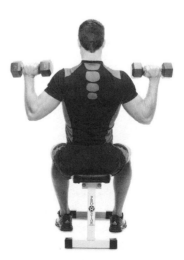

The subjects were able to maintain the level of fitness they had achieved with the 12-week program by working out just 1 day a week. For you, that means starting at the same place you were before time sidetracked you.

Not blowing off exercise completely for the week also keeps your muscles from forgetting what they have to do the next time you exercise. Deep within your muscles, tendons, and joints are a series of nerves, or *proprioceptors,* that help stabilize your body as you exercise. Avoiding exercise entirely for the week can cause them to become less effective, leaving you with less coordination and fewer results the next time you exercise. Getting in at least a day of exercise can keep these sensory nerves sharp, so your posture stays perfect down the road.

HERE'S HOW TO TWEAK YOUR WEEK

There are thousands of exercises you can use to build a better body. But with only 1 day in your schedule, it's essential that you stick with the basic exercises, no matter what your goals are.

Each of these routines—except for the shorter "lean-body" programs—will ask you to do a full-body routine that hits all your major muscle groups in the same workout. I've chosen the most-effective exercises for building muscle for each body part, incorporating compound exercises that force more of your muscles to work together.

For you, that means faster results . . . in less time.

Same Time, More Results

WATCH WHERE YOU PUT YOUR HANDS.

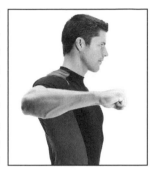

Maintain a straight wrist when holding any weight, cable handle, resistance band, or the like. This keeps the center of your palm in line with your forearm, transferring the weight directly through your arms. Conversely, if you bend your wrists back or curl them forward, it forces your wrists to bear most of the pressure with nothing behind them to back them up. This takes power out of the movement, leaving you lifting less weight than you could be. It also torques the ligaments, tendons, and joints within your wrists, placing them at risk of immediate injury or long-term damage.

To get in the habit of how your wrists should look—and feel—when they're in the right position, do this trick before starting any exercise. Pretend you're punching something, pull back your arm, then look at your wrist. Your fist and wrist should be in a straight line with your forearm. Keep that form—and feel—in mind as you exercise. If you can't maintain that perfect form as you exercise, try decreasing the amount of weight you're using. (It's okay not to maintain straight wrists when doing wrist curls and extensions—that's the nature of the exercise.)

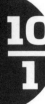

10 Minutes/1 Day a Week

Your Instant LEAN-BODY Plan!

1 minute of low-intensity cardiovascular exercise

8 minutes of high-intensity cardio

1 minute of low-intensity cardio

Your Instant POWER Plan!

Rest 45 seconds between sets.

- 3 sets/**Squat** (6–8 reps)
- 3 sets/**Deadlift** (6–8 reps)
- 2 sets/**Bench press** (6–8 reps)

Your Instant MUSCLE Plan!

Rest 30 seconds between sets.

1 set/**Squat** (8–12 reps)

1 set/**Lunge** (8–12 reps)

1 set/**Bench press** (8–12 reps)

1 set/**Bent-over row** (8–12 reps)

1 set/**Seated shoulder press** (8–12 reps)

1 set/**Biceps curl** (8–12 reps)

1 set/**Seated triceps extension** (8–12 reps)

1 set/**Crunch** (done until failure—i.e., you can't do any more)

10 Minutes/1 Day a Week

Your Instant **COMPLETE-BODY** Plan!

Rest 30 seconds between sets.

1 set/**Squat**
(8–12 reps)

1 set/**Lunge**
(8–12 reps)

1 set/**Bench press**
(8–12 reps)

1 set/**Bent-over row**
(8–12 reps)

1 set/**Seated shoulder press**
(8–12 reps)

1 set/**Biceps curl**
(8–12 reps)

1 set/**Seated triceps extension**
(8–12 reps)

1 set/**Crunch**
(done until failure)

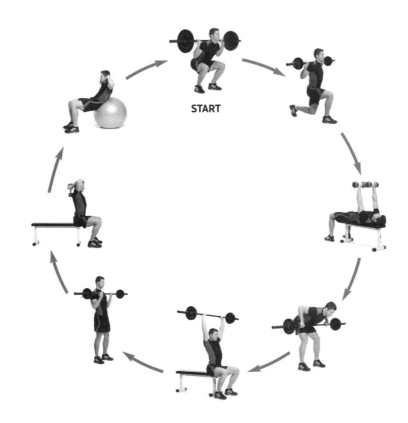

START

20 Minutes/1 Day a Week

20/1

Your Instant LEAN-BODY Plan!

2 minutes of low-intensity cardiovascular exercise

16 minutes of medium-intensity cardio

2 minutes of low-intensity cardio

Your Instant POWER Plan!

Rest 60 seconds between sets.

- ⚡ 4 sets/**Squat** (6–8 reps)
- ⚡ 3 sets/**Deadlift** (6–8 reps)
- ⚡ 3 sets/**Power clean** (6–8 reps)
- ⚡ 3 sets/**Bench press** (6–8 reps)

Your Instant MUSCLE Plan!

Rest 30 seconds between sets.

3 sets/**Squat** (8–12 reps)

2 sets/**Lunge** (8–12 reps)

2 sets/**Bench press** (8–12 reps)

2 sets/**Bent-over row** (8–12 reps)

2 sets/**Seated shoulder press** (8–12 reps)

2 sets/**Biceps curl** (8–12 reps)

2 sets/**Seated triceps extension** (8–12 reps)

1 set/**Crunch** (done until failure)

1 set/**Reverse crunch** (done until failure)

Your Instant COMPLETE-BODY Plan!

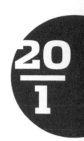

Rest 30 seconds between sets.

2 sets/**Squat**
(8–12 reps; 6–8 reps)

2 sets/**Deadlift**
(8–12 reps; 6–8 reps)

2 sets/**Lunge**
(8–12 reps; 6–8 reps)

2 sets/**Bench press**
(8–12 reps; 6–8 reps)

2 sets/**Bent-over row**
(8–12 reps; 6–8 reps)

2 sets/**Seated shoulder press**
(8–12 reps; 6–8 reps)

2 sets/**Biceps curl**
(8–12 reps; 6–8 reps)

2 sets/**Seated triceps extension**
(8–12 reps; 6–8 reps)

1 set/**Crunch**
(done until failure)

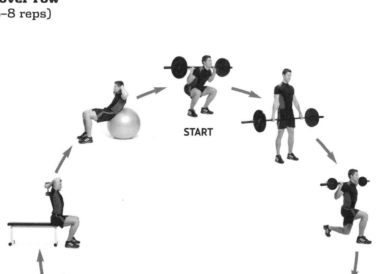

START

30 Minutes/1 Day a Week

30/1

Your Instant LEAN-BODY Plan!

Rest 15 seconds between sets.

2 minutes of low-intensity cardiovascular exercise

1 set/**Squat** (12–15 reps)

1 set/**Lunge** (12–15 reps)

1 set/**Bench press** (12–15 reps)

1 set/**Bent-over row** (12–15 reps)

1 set/**Seated shoulder press** (12–15 reps)

1 set/**Biceps curl** (12–15 reps)

1 set/**Seated triceps extension** (12–15 reps)

1 set/**Crunch** (done until failure)

16 minutes of medium-intensity cardio

2 minutes of low-intensity cardio

Your Instant POWER Plan!

Rest 60 seconds between sets.

⚡ 4 sets/**Squat** (6–8 reps) ⚡ 3 sets/**Bench press** (6–8 reps)

⚡ 4 sets/**Deadlift** (6–8 reps) ⚡ 3 sets/**Push press** (6–8 reps)

⚡ 3 sets/**Power clean** (6–8 reps) ⚡ 3 sets/**Bent-over row** (6–8 reps)

Your Instant MUSCLE Plan!

Rest 30 seconds between sets.

4 sets/**Squat** (8–12 reps)

4 sets/**Deadlift** (8–12 reps)

3 sets/**Bench press** (8–12 reps)

3 sets/**Bent-over row** (8–12 reps)

3 sets/**Seated shoulder press** (8–12 reps)

3 sets/**Biceps curl** (8–12 reps)

3 sets/**Seated triceps extension** (8–12 reps)

1 set/**Crunch** (done until failure)

1 set/**Reverse crunch** (done until failure)

30 Minutes/1 Day a Week

Your Instant COMPLETE-BODY Plan!

Rest 30 seconds between sets.

3 sets/**Squat**
(12–15 reps; 8–12 reps; 6–8 reps)

3 sets/**Deadlift**
(12–15 reps; 8–12 reps; 6–8 reps)

3 sets/**Lunge**
(12–15 reps; 8–12 reps; 6–8 reps)

3 sets/**Bench press**
(12–15 reps; 8–12 reps; 6–8 reps)

3 sets/**Bent-over row**
(12–15 reps; 8–12 reps; 6–8 reps)

3 sets/**Seated shoulder press**
(12–15 reps; 8–12 reps; 6–8 reps)

2 sets/**Biceps curl**
(8–12 reps; 6–8 reps)

2 sets/**Seated triceps extension**
(8–12 reps; 6–8 reps)

1 set/**Crunch**
(done until failure)

1 set/**Reverse crunch**
(done until failure)

1 set/**V-up with a twist**
(done until failure)

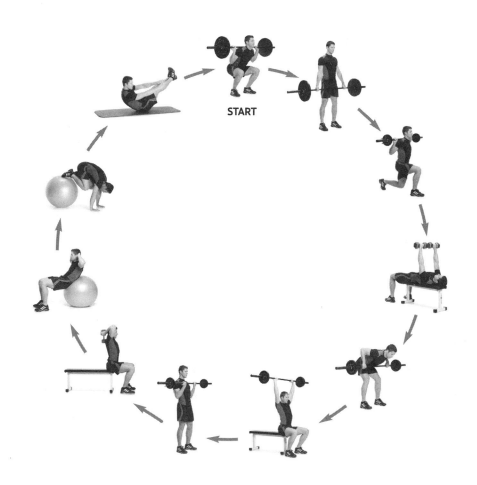

START

45 Minutes/1 Day a Week

45/1

Your Instant LEAN-BODY Plan!

Rest 15 seconds between sets.

2 minutes of low-intensity cardiovascular exercise

2 sets/**Squat** (12–15 reps)

2 sets/**Lunge** (12–15 reps)

2 sets/**Bench press** (12–15 reps)

2 sets/**One-arm row** (12–15 reps)

2 sets/**Seated shoulder press** (12–15 reps)

2 sets/**Biceps curl** (12–15 reps)

2 sets/**Seated triceps extension** (12–15 reps)

1 set/**Crunch** (done until failure)

1 set/**Reverse crunch** (done until failure)

20 minutes of medium-intensity cardio

3 minutes of low-intensity cardio

Your Instant POWER Plan!

Rest 90 seconds between sets.

⚡ 5 sets/**Squat** (6–8 reps)

⚡ 4 sets/**Deadlift** (6–8 reps)

⚡ 4 sets/**Bench press** (6–8 reps)

⚡ 3 sets/**Push press** (6–8 reps)

⚡ 3 sets/**Bent-over row** (6–8 reps)

⚡ 2 sets/**Biceps curl** (6–8 reps)

⚡ 2 sets/**Dip** (6–8 reps)

Your Instant MUSCLE Plan!

Rest 45 seconds between sets.

4 sets/**Squat** (8–12 reps)

4 sets/**Deadlift** (8–12 reps)

4 sets/**Bench press** (8–12 reps)

3 sets/**Incline press** (8–12 reps)

4 sets/**Bent-over row** (8–12 reps)

3 sets/**Seated shoulder press** (8–12 reps)

3 sets/**Biceps curl** (8–12 reps)

3 sets/**Seated triceps extension** (8–12 reps)

1 set/**Crunch** (done until failure)

1 set/**Reverse crunch** (done until failure)

45 Minutes/1 Day a Week

Your Instant COMPLETE-BODY Plan!

45/1

Rest 45 seconds between sets.

4 sets/**Squat**
(12–15 reps; 8–12 reps; 6–8 reps; 6–8 reps)

4 sets/**Deadlift**
(12–15 reps; 8–12 reps; 6–8 reps; 6–8 reps)

3 sets/**Lunge**
(12–15 reps; 8–12 reps; 6–8 reps)

3 sets/**Bench press**
(12–15 reps; 8–12 reps; 6–8 reps)

3 sets/**Bent-over row**
(12–15 reps; 8–12 reps; 6–8 reps)

3 sets/**Seated shoulder press**
(12–15 reps; 8–12 reps; 6–8 reps)

3 sets/**Lateral raise**
(12–15 reps; 8–12 reps; 6–8 reps)

2 sets/**Biceps curl**
(8–12 reps; 6–8 reps)

2 sets/**Seated triceps extension**
(8–12 reps; 6–8 reps)

1 set/**Crunch**
(done until failure)

1 set/**Reverse crunch**
(done until failure)

1 set/**V-up with a twist**
(done until failure)

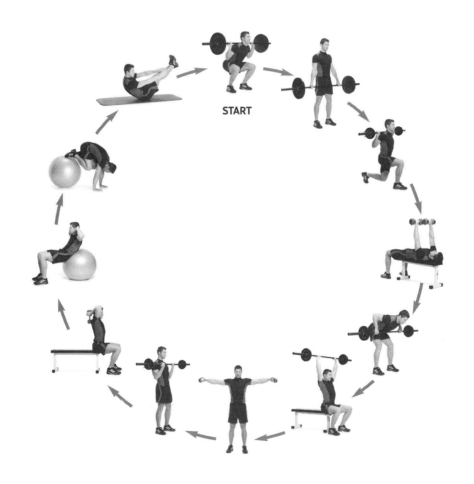

START

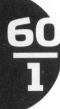

60 Minutes/1 Day a Week

Your Instant LEAN-BODY Plan!

Rest 15 seconds between sets.

2 minutes of low-intensity cardiovascular exercise

3 sets/**Squat** (12–15 reps)

3 sets/**Lunge** (12–15 reps)

3 sets/**Bench press** (12–15 reps)

3 sets/**One-arm row** (12–15 reps)

3 sets/**Seated shoulder press** (12–15 reps)

2 sets/**Biceps curl** (12–15 reps)

2 sets/**Seated triceps extension** (12–15 reps)

1 set/**Crunch** (done until failure)

1 set/**Reverse crunch** (done until failure)

30 minutes of medium-intensity cardio

3 minutes of low-intensity cardio

Your Instant POWER Plan!

Rest 2 minutes between sets.

⚡ 5 sets/**Squat** (6–8 reps)

⚡ 5 sets/**Deadlift** (6–8 reps)

⚡ 4 sets/**Bench press** (6–8 reps)

⚡ 3 sets/**Push press** (6–8 reps)

⚡ 3 sets/**Bent-over row** (6–8 reps)

⚡ 2 sets/**Biceps curl** (6–8 reps)

⚡ 2 sets/**Dip** (6–8 reps)

Your Instant MUSCLE Plan!

Rest 60 seconds between sets.

4 sets/**Deadlift** (8–12 reps)

3 sets/**Lunge** (8–12 reps)

3 sets/**Bench press** (8–12 reps)

3 sets/**Incline press** (8–12 reps)

3 sets/**Bent-over row** (8–12 reps)

3 sets/**Lat pulldown** (8–12 reps)

3 sets/**Seated shoulder press** (8–12 reps)

2 sets/**Lateral raise** (8–12 reps)

3 sets/**Biceps curl** (8–12 reps)

3 sets/**Seated triceps extension** (8–12 reps)

1 set/**Crunch** (done until failure)

1 set/**Reverse crunch** (done until failure)

Your Instant COMPLETE-BODY Plan!

60/1

Rest 60 seconds between sets.

4 sets/**Squat**
(12–15 reps; 8–12 reps; 6–8 reps; 6–8 reps)

4 sets/**Deadlift**
(12–15 reps; 8–12 reps; 6–8 reps; 6–8 reps)

3 sets/**Lunge**
(12–15 reps; 8–12 reps; 6–8 reps)

3 sets/**Bench press**
(12–15 reps; 8–12 reps; 6–8 reps)

3 sets/**Incline press**
(12–15 reps; 8–12 reps; 6–8 reps)

3 sets/**Bent-over row**
(12–15 reps; 8–12 reps; 6–8 reps)

3 sets/**Lat pulldown**
(12–15 reps; 8–12 reps; 6–8 reps)

3 sets/**Seated shoulder press**
(12–15 reps; 8–12 reps; 6–8 reps)

3 sets/**Lateral raise**
(12–15 reps; 8–12 reps; 6–8 reps)

2 sets/**Biceps curl**
(8–12 reps; 6–8 reps)

2 sets/**Seated triceps extension**
(8–12 reps; 6–8 reps)

1 set/**Crunch**
(done until failure)

1 set/**Reverse crunch**
(done until failure)

1 set/**V-up with a twist**
(done until failure)

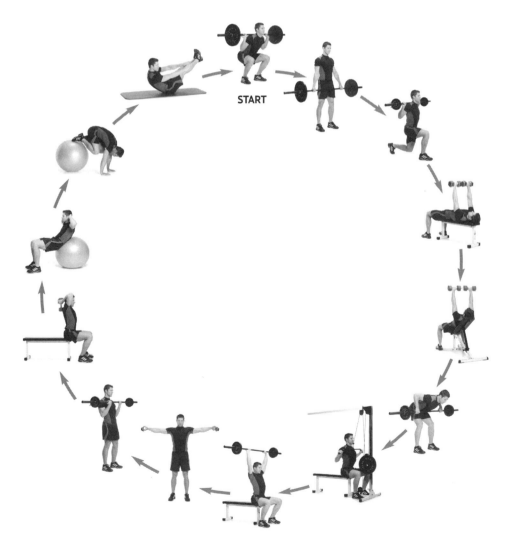

START

I Have Only 2 Days a Week

Why Just 2 Days Is Still Okay

It may still be less than what's recommended, but there's a lot to be said for taking the time to at least "do two."

If you can't fit 3 days into your schedule, then aiming for 2 instead is more productive than most people realize. Research has proven that exercising twice a week for as little as 20 minutes a session can add 3 pounds of muscle and burn off more than 4 pounds of fat in just 8 weeks.

In fact, research has shown that strength training twice a week is nearly 90 percent as effective as 3 days a week for building strength and improving the size and shape of your muscles. That means if you've been seeing incredible results from a 3-day-a-week workout schedule, blowing off 1 day and making it a 2-day affair will leave your workouts only 10 percent less effective.

TIME TWEAKS!

Spend Less Time . . . Looking at Things You Shouldn't Be!

Bending your neck when lifting weights, just to cop a peek to see who may be staring at you, places you at risk of more than a cold stare back. Almost every upper-body exercise, whether it's a curl, a press, or a pulldown, requires your spinal erectors to help stabilize your back as you lift. These muscles end at your neck, where they stay stiff from contracting every time you lift. Looking around is like pulling on a rubber band that's already stretched as far as it can go. Moving in any direction can cause you to strain muscle tissues or—even worse—place stress on the disks within your spine.

To avoid this, always look straight ahead when you're exercising, always keep your neck in line with your back, and keep your head up. Imagine there's a string attached to your head and someone is pulling up on it. If you need to watch your form—or someone else in the gym—use a mirror instead, to see the big picture without having to crane your neck.

TIME TWEAKS!

Spend More Time . . . Exercising Even When You Have No Weights!

When you can't find time for the weight room, try a few isometric moves instead. Pushing and pulling against an immovable object—mimicking some of the "anytime" exercises in this book—can tone and strengthen muscles almost as effectively as weight training can. Find a sturdy wall, or even the sides of a table or desk, and gently push or pull against it, increasing your effort slowly (to make sure the ob-

ject remains in place as you go) until you're exerting all your effort. Hold this position for 6 to 8 seconds, then rest and repeat the drill two or three times.

To strengthen your arms, find a sturdy desk and grab the edge of it as if it were a bar. To work your biceps, you can place your hands flat underneath the edge of the desk and gently press upward as if you were trying to curl it up. Hold this position for 6 to 8 seconds—your biceps should contract as you maintain the pose—then rest and repeat the move two or three more times. Likewise, placing your palms on top of the desk and pressing

downward mimics a triceps push-down, to work your triceps.

To work your upper body in a pinch, stand next to a sturdy door, grab the door handle, and slowly pull until you feel your back muscles tighten. Hold for 6 to 8 seconds, gently release, and repeat two or three more times. To strengthen your chest, shut the door and press your hands against it—elbows bent—and press as hard as you can for 6 to 8 seconds. The better you understand the 48 "anytime" exercises, the easier it will be to mimic some of them using no equipment at all when you have no other option.

Here's How to Tweak Your Week

The same rules that apply to exercising once a week apply to the twice-a-week schedule. Both days, you'll be asked to do a full-body program that works all your muscle groups in one shot, using more multijoint, compound exercises that develop more muscle fibers in the shortest period of time. However, it's important to remember which days you're allowed to exercise.

For some of you, the 2-day-a-week schedule may be the result of having only the weekend to exercise. If your game plan was to use these 2-day programs on Saturday *and* Sunday, you're forgetting something very important that I mentioned earlier in this book. Your muscles need at least 48 hours to recover from the stresses you're placing them under when you exercise. Doing any of the fol-

lowing routines on a Saturday and Sunday schedule doesn't leave them enough time to rest and rebuild. You need to place *at least 1 day* between these two workouts.

Ideally, you should try to space them evenly throughout the week (Monday and Thursday, for example) instead of lumping them closer to each other (Monday and Wednesday), which leaves a longer rest period between workouts. Exercising on a Monday/Wednesday schedule means that your body has to wait 5 days between Wednesday and the following Monday.

Now that you know the rules, it's time to get rolling. Whether you're using these routines because you're strapped for time or because you're still easing your way into exercise, these four "instant plans" will ensure that your mind and muscles are ready for the ride ahead.

10 Minutes/2 Days a Week

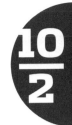

Your Instant LEAN-BODY Plan!

Both Days

1 minute of low-intensity cardiovascular exercise

8 minutes of high-intensity cardio

1 minute of low-intensity cardio

Your Instant POWER Plan!

Both Days (Rest 45 seconds between sets)

⚡ 3 sets/**Squat** (6–8 reps)

⚡ 3 sets/**Deadlift** (6–8 reps)

⚡ 2 sets/**Bench press** (6–8 reps)

Your Instant MUSCLE Plan!

Both Days (Rest 30 seconds between sets)

1 set/**Squat** (8–12 reps)

1 set/**Lunge** (8–12 reps)

1 set/**Bench press** (8–12 reps)

1 set/**Bent-over row** (8–12 reps)

1 set/**Seated shoulder press** (8–12 reps)

1 set/**Biceps curl** (8–12 reps)

1 set/**Seated triceps extension** (8–12 reps)

1 set/**Crunch** (done until failure—
i.e., you can't do any more)

10 Minutes/2 Days a Week

▶ Your Instant **COMPLETE-BODY** Plan!

10
2

Day 1 (Rest 30 seconds between sets)

1 set/**Squat**
(8–12 reps)

1 set/**Lunge**
(8–12 reps)

1 set/**Bench press**
(8–12 reps)

1 set/**Bent-over row**
(8–12 reps)

1 set/**Seated shoulder press**
(8–12 reps)

1 set/**Biceps curl**
(8–12 reps)

1 set/**Seated triceps extension**
(8–12 reps)

1 set/**Crunch**
(done until failure)

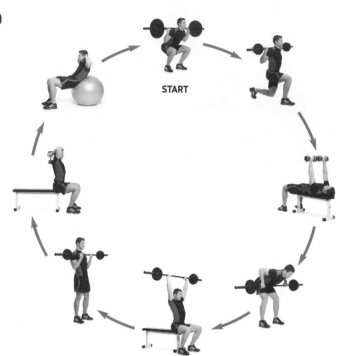

- -

Day 2 (Rest 45 seconds between sets)

3 sets/**Squat**
(6–8 reps)

3 sets/**Deadlift**
(6–8 reps)

2 sets/**Bench press**
(6–8 reps)

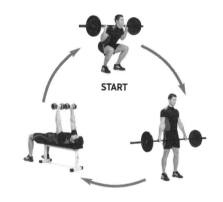

20 Minutes/2 Days a Week

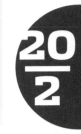

Your Instant LEAN-BODY Plan!

Both Days

2 minutes of low-intensity cardiovascular exercise

16 minutes of medium-intensity cardio

2 minutes of low-intensity cardio

Your Instant POWER Plan!

Both Days (Rest 60 seconds between sets)

⚡ 4 sets/**Squat** (6–8 reps)

⚡ 3 sets/**Deadlift** (6–8 reps)

⚡ 3 sets/**Power clean** (6–8 reps)

⚡ 3 sets/**Bench press** (6–8 reps)

Your Instant MUSCLE Plan!

Both Days (Rest 30 seconds between sets)

3 sets/**Squat** (8–12 reps)

2 sets/**Lunge** (8–12 reps)

2 sets/**Bench press** (8–12 reps)

2 sets/**Bent-over row** (8–12 reps)

2 sets/**Seated shoulder press** (8–12 reps)

2 sets/**Biceps curl** (8–12 reps)

2 sets/**Seated triceps extension** (8–12 reps)

1 set/**Crunch** (done until failure)

1 set/**Reverse crunch** (done until failure)

20 Minutes/2 Days a Week

Your Instant COMPLETE-BODY Plan!

Day 1 (Rest 30 seconds between sets)

2 sets/**Squat**
(8–12 reps; 6–8 reps)

2 sets/**Deadlift**
(8–12 reps; 6–8 reps)

2 sets/**Lunge**
(8–12 reps; 6–8 reps)

2 sets/**Bench press**
(8–12 reps; 6–8 reps)

2 sets/**Bent-over row**
(8–12 reps; 6–8 reps)

2 sets/**Seated shoulder press**
(8–12 reps; 6–8 reps)

2 sets/**Biceps curl**
(8–12 reps; 6–8 reps)

2 sets/**Seated triceps extension**
(8–12 reps; 6–8 reps)

1 set/**Crunch**
(done until failure)

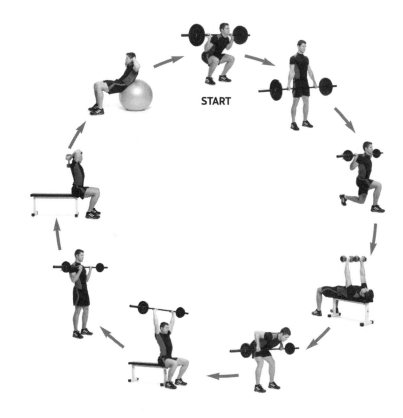

START

Day 2 (Rest 30 seconds between sets)

2 sets/**Front squat**
(12–15 reps; 8–12 reps)

2 sets/**Deadlift**
(12–15 reps; 8–12 reps)

2 sets/**Reverse lunge**
(12–15 reps; 8–12 reps)

2 sets/**Bench press**
(12–15 reps; 8–12 reps)

2 sets/**Bent-over row**
(12–15 reps; 8–12 reps)

2 sets/**Seated shoulder press**
(12–15 reps; 8–12 reps)

2 sets/**Biceps curl**
(12–15 reps; 8–12 reps)

2 sets/**Dip**
(12–15 reps; 8–12 reps)

2 sets/**Reverse crunch**
(each set done until failure)

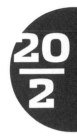

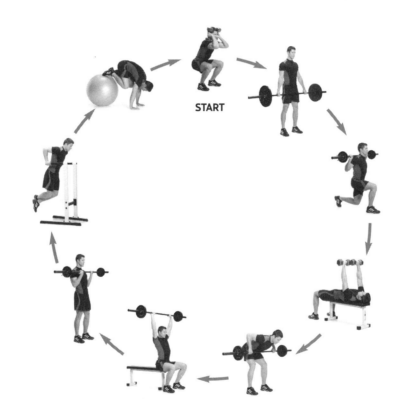

START

30 Minutes/2 Days a Week

30/2

Your Instant LEAN-BODY Plan!

Both Days (Rest 15 seconds between sets)

2 minutes of low-intensity cardiovascular exercise

1 set/**Squat** (12–15 reps)

1 set/**Lunge** (12–15 reps)

1 set/**Bench press** (12–15 reps)

1 set/**Bent-over row** (12–15 reps)

1 set/**Seated shoulder press** (12–15 reps)

1 set/**Biceps curl** (12–15 reps)

1 set/**Seated triceps extension** (12–15 reps)

1 set/**Crunch** (done until failure)

16 minutes of medium-intensity cardio

2 minutes of low-intensity cardio

Your Instant POWER Plan!

Both Days (Rest 60 seconds between sets)

4 sets/**Squat** (6–8 reps)

4 sets/**Deadlift** (6–8 reps)

3 sets/**Power clean** (6–8 reps)

3 sets/**Bench press** (6–8 reps)

3 sets/**Push press** (6–8 reps)

3 sets/**Bent-over row** (6–8 reps)

Your Instant MUSCLE Plan!

Both Days (Rest 30 seconds between sets)

4 sets/**Squat** (8–12 reps)

4 sets/**Deadlift** (8–12 reps)

3 sets/**Bench press** (8–12 reps)

3 sets/**Bent-over row** (8–12 reps)

3 sets/**Seated shoulder press** (8–12 reps)

3 sets/**Biceps curl** (8–12 reps)

3 sets/**Seated triceps extension** (8–12 reps)

1 set/**Crunch** (done until failure)

1 set/**Reverse crunch** (done until failure)

30/2

TIME TWEAKS!

Spend More Time . . . Remembering What's Behind You!

If you think it's easiest just to drop exercises from any of these programs because you don't have much time—or because you don't care as much about the muscles they work—think again! You're about to fall into the biggest trap that many beginning to intermediate exercisers fall victim to—a trap that leaves them quitting exercise before it can do its job.

Many exercisers focus solely on the muscles they can see in the mirror, ignoring the ones the rest of us have to look at. Neglecting the muscles that are behind you (the neck, rear shoulders, lower back, butt, hamstrings, and calves) is a mistake that can leave you injury-prone and weaker over time.

Strengthening the muscles in front tightens them, causing them to pull on the weaker muscles that are behind them. The result can create muscle imbalances that shift your spine, knees, and elbows out of alignment, increasing your

chances of injury. It can also leave you looking out of proportion and give you a hunched back and shoulders.

All of the routines in this book are designed to ensure an even body, but if you do ever decide to go "off the menu," make sure that your workout divides itself equally between the muscles in front and the muscles in back. For every front-muscle exercise you do, be sure to add an exercise that works the muscles located right in back of it—for example, do a lower-back exercise for every abdominal exercise.

30 Minutes/2 Days a Week

Your Instant **COMPLETE-BODY** Plan!

Day 1 (Rest 30 seconds between sets)

3 sets/**Squat**
(12–15 reps; 8–12 reps; 6–8 reps)

3 sets/**Deadlift**
(12–15 reps; 8–12 reps; 6–8 reps)

3 sets/**Lunge**
(12–15 reps; 8–12 reps; 6–8 reps)

3 sets/**Bench press**
(12–15 reps; 8–12 reps; 6–8 reps)

3 sets/**Bent-over row**
(12–15 reps; 8–12 reps; 6–8 reps)

3 sets/**Seated shoulder press**
(12–15 reps; 8–12 reps; 6–8 reps)

2 sets/**Biceps curl**
(8–12 reps; 6–8 reps)

2 sets/**Seated triceps extension**
(8–12 reps; 6–8 reps)

1 set/**Crunch**
(done until failure)

1 set/**Reverse crunch**
(done until failure)

1 set/**V-up with a twist**
(done until failure)

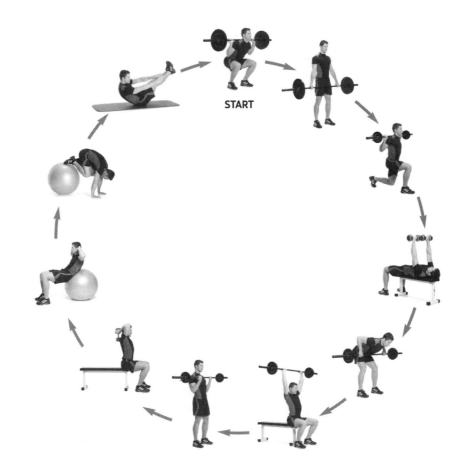

START

Day 2 (Rest 30 seconds between sets)

3 sets/**Front squat**
(12–15 reps; 8–12 reps; 6–8 reps)

3 sets/**Reverse lunge**
(12–15 reps; 8–12 reps; 6–8 reps)

3 sets/**Deadlift**
(12–15 reps; 8–12 reps; 6–8 reps)

3 sets/**Bench press**
(12–15 reps; 8–12 reps; 6–8 reps)

3 sets/**Lat pulldown**
(12–15 reps; 8–12 reps; 6–8 reps)

3 sets/**Push press**
(12–15 reps; 8–12 reps; 6–8 reps)

2 sets/**Hammer curl**
(8–12 reps; 6–8 reps)

2 sets/**Triceps pushdown**
(8–12 reps; 6–8 reps)

1 set/**Twisting crunch**
(done until failure)

1 set/**Twisting toe touch**
(done until failure)

1 set/**Side raise**
(done until failure)

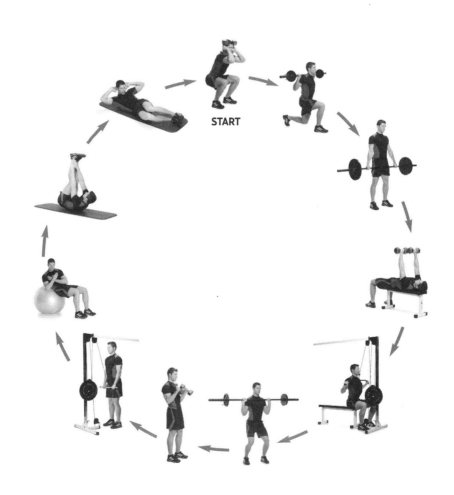

START

45 Minutes/2 Days a Week

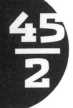

Your Instant LEAN-BODY Plan!

Both Days (Rest 15 seconds between sets)

2 minutes of low-intensity cardiovascular exercise

2 sets/**Squat** (12–15 reps)

2 sets/**Lunge** (12–15 reps)

2 sets/**Bench press** (12–15 reps)

2 sets/**One-arm row** (12–15 reps)

2 sets/**Seated shoulder press** (12–15 reps)

2 sets/**Biceps curl** (12–15 reps)

2 sets/**Seated triceps extension** (12–15 reps)

1 set/**Crunch** (done until failure)

1 set/**Reverse crunch** (done until failure)

20 minutes of medium-intensity cardio

3 minutes of low-intensity cardio

Your Instant POWER Plan!

Both Days (Rest 90 seconds between sets)

5 sets/**Squat** (6–8 reps)

4 sets/**Deadlift** (6–8 reps)

4 sets/**Bench press** (6–8 reps)

3 sets/**Push press** (6–8 reps)

3 sets/**Bent-over row** (6–8 reps)

2 sets/**Biceps curl** (6–8 reps)

2 sets/**Dip** (6–8 reps)

Your Instant MUSCLE Plan!

Both Days (Rest 45 seconds between sets)

4 sets/**Squat** (8–12 reps)

4 sets/**Deadlift** (8–12 reps)

4 sets/**Bench press** (8–12 reps)

3 sets/**Incline press** (8–12 reps)

4 sets/**Bent-over row** (8–12 reps)

3 sets/**Seated shoulder press** (8–12 reps)

3 sets/**Biceps curl** (8–12 reps)

3 sets/**Seated triceps extension** (8–12 reps)

1 set/**Crunch** (done until failure)

1 set/**Reverse crunch** (done until failure)

45/2

45 Minutes/2 Days a Week

▶ Your Instant **COMPLETE-BODY** Plan!

45/2

Day 1 (Rest 45 seconds between sets)

4 sets/Squat
(12–15 reps; 8–12 reps; 6–8 reps; 6–8 reps)

4 sets/Deadlift
(12–15 reps; 8–12 reps; 6–8 reps; 6–8 reps)

2 sets/Lunge
(12–15 reps; 8–12 reps)

3 sets/Bench press
(12–15 reps; 8–12 reps; 6–8 reps)

3 sets/Bent-over row
(12–15 reps; 8–12 reps; 6–8 reps)

3 sets/Seated shoulder press
(12–15 reps; 8–12 reps; 6–8 reps)

3 sets/Lateral raise
(12–15 reps; 8–12 reps; 6–8 reps)

2 sets/Biceps curl
(8–12 reps; 6–8 reps)

2 sets/Seated triceps extension
(8–12 reps; 6–8 reps)

1 set/Crunch
(done until failure)

1 set/Reverse crunch
(done until failure)

1 set/V-up with a twist
(done until failure)

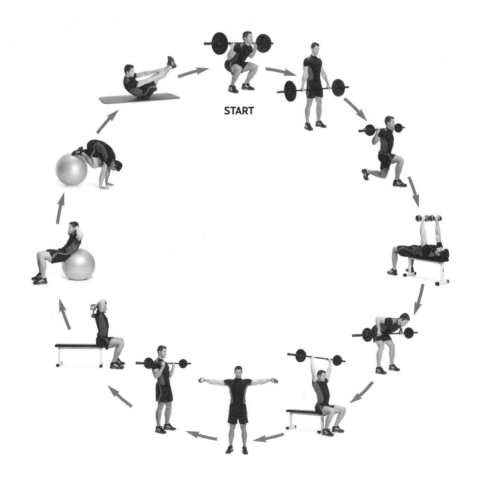

START

Day 2 (Rest 45 seconds between sets)

4 sets/**Squat**
(12–15 reps; 8–12 reps; 6–8 reps; 6–8 reps)

4 sets/**Deadlift**
(12–15 reps; 8–12 reps; 6–8 reps; 6–8 reps)

2 sets/**Reverse lunge**
(12–15 reps; 8–12 reps)

3 sets/**Bench press**
(12–15 reps; 8–12 reps; 6–8 reps)

3 sets/**Bent-over row**
(12–15 reps; 8–12 reps; 6–8 reps)

3 sets/**Seated shoulder press**
(12–15 reps; 8–12 reps; 6–8 reps)

3 sets/**Bent-over reverse raise**
(12–15 reps; 8–12 reps; 6–8 reps)

2 sets/**Hammer curl**
(8–12 reps; 6–8 reps)

2 sets/**Dip**
(8–12 reps; 6–8 reps)

1 set/**Twisting crunch**
(done until failure)

1 set/**Twisting leg thrust**
(done until failure)

1 set/**Twisting toe touch**
(done until failure)

45/2

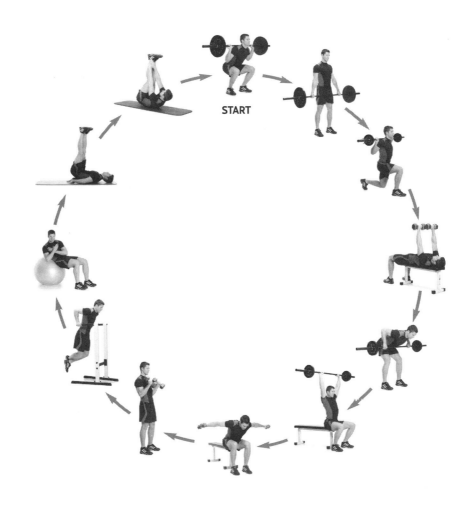

START

60 Minutes/2 Days a Week

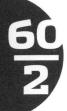

Your Instant LEAN-BODY Plan!

Both Days (Rest 15 seconds between sets)

2 minutes of low-intensity cardiovascular exercise

3 sets/**Squat** (12–15 reps)

3 sets/**Lunge** (12–15 reps)

3 sets/**Bench press** (12–15 reps)

3 sets/**One-arm row** (12–15 reps)

3 sets/**Seated shoulder press** (12–15 reps)

2 sets/**Biceps curl** (12–15 reps)

2 sets/**Seated triceps extension** (12–15 reps)

1 set/**Crunch** (done until failure)

1 set/**Reverse crunch** (done until failure)

30 minutes of medium-intensity cardio

3 minutes of low-intensity cardio

Your Instant POWER Plan!

Day 1 (Rest 2 minutes between sets)

- 5 sets/**Squat** (6–8 reps)
- 5 sets/**Deadlift** (6–8 reps)
- 4 sets/**Bench press** (6–8 reps)
- 3 sets/**Push press** (6–8 reps)
- 3 sets/**Bent-over row** (6–8 reps)
- 2 sets/**Biceps curl** (6–8 reps)
- 2 sets/**Dip** (6–8 reps)

Day 2 (Rest 2 minutes between sets)

- 5 sets/**Squat** (6–8 reps)
- 5 sets/**Deadlift** (6–8 reps)
- 4 sets/**Bench press** (6–8 reps)
- 3 sets/**Seated shoulder press** (6–8 reps)
- 3 sets/**One-arm row** (6–8 reps)
- 2 sets/**Biceps curl** (6–8 reps)
- 2 sets/**Dip** (6–8 reps)

Your Instant MUSCLE Plan!

Both Days (Rest 60 seconds between sets)

4 sets/**Deadlift** (8–12 reps)

3 sets/**Lunge** (8–12 reps)

3 sets/**Bench press** (8–12 reps)

3 sets/**Incline press** (8–12 reps)

3 sets/**Bent-over row** (8–12 reps)

3 sets/**Lat pulldown** (8–12 reps)

3 sets/**Seated shoulder press** (8–12 reps)

2 sets/**Lateral raise** (8–12 reps)

3 sets/**Biceps curl** (8–12 reps)

3 sets/**Seated triceps extension** (8–12 reps)

1 set/**Crunch** (done until failure)

1 set/**Reverse crunch** (done until failure)

60/2

60 Minutes/2 Days a Week

Your Instant COMPLETE-BODY Plan!

60/2

Day 1 (Rest 60 seconds between sets)

4 sets/**Squat**
(12–15 reps; 8–12 reps; 6–8 reps; 6–8 reps)

4 sets/**Deadlift**
(12–15 reps; 8–12 reps; 6–8 reps; 6–8 reps)

3 sets/**Lunge**
(12–15 reps; 8–12 reps; 6–8 reps)

3 sets/**Bench press**
(12–15 reps; 8–12 reps; 6–8 reps)

3 sets/**Incline press**
(12–15 reps; 8–12 reps; 6–8 reps)

3 sets/**Bent-over row**
(12–15 reps; 8–12 reps; 6–8 reps)

3 sets/**Lat pulldown**
(12–15 reps; 8–12 reps; 6–8 reps)

3 sets/**Seated shoulder press**
(12–15 reps; 8–12 reps; 6–8 reps)

3 sets/**Lateral raise**
(12–15 reps; 8–12 reps; 6–8 reps)

2 sets/**Biceps curl**
(8–12 reps; 6–8 reps)

2 sets/**Seated triceps extension**
(8–12 reps; 6–8 reps)

1 set/**Crunch**
(done until failure)

1 set/**Reverse crunch**
(done until failure)

1 set/**V-up with a twist**
(done until failure)

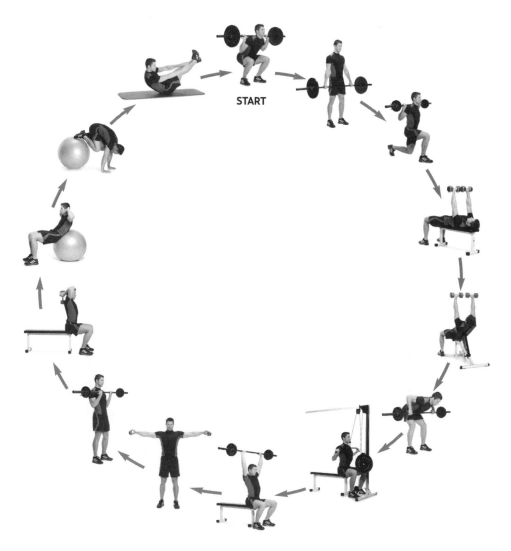

START

Day 2 (Rest 60 seconds between sets)

4 sets/**Squat**
(12–15 reps; 8–12 reps; 6–8 reps; 6–8 reps)

4 sets/**Deadlift**
(12–15 reps; 8–12 reps; 6–8 reps; 6–8 reps)

3 sets/**Reverse lunge**
(12–15 reps; 8–12 reps; 6–8 reps)

3 sets/**Bench press**
(12–15 reps; 8–12 reps; 6–8 reps)

3 sets/**Incline fly**
(12–15 reps; 8–12 reps; 6–8 reps)

3 sets/**One-arm row**
(12–15 reps; 8–12 reps; 6–8 reps)

3 sets/**Close-grip pulldown**
(12–15 reps; 8–12 reps; 6–8 reps)

3 sets/**Seated shoulder press**
(12–15 reps; 8–12 reps; 6–8 reps)

3 sets/**Lateral raise**
(12–15 reps; 8–12 reps; 6–8 reps)

2 sets/**Hammer curl**
(8–12 reps; 6–8 reps)

2 sets/**Dip**
(8–12 reps; 6–8 reps)

1 set/**Twisting crunch**
(done until failure)

1 set/**Twisting leg thrust**
(done until failure)

1 set/**Twisting toe touch**
(done until failure)

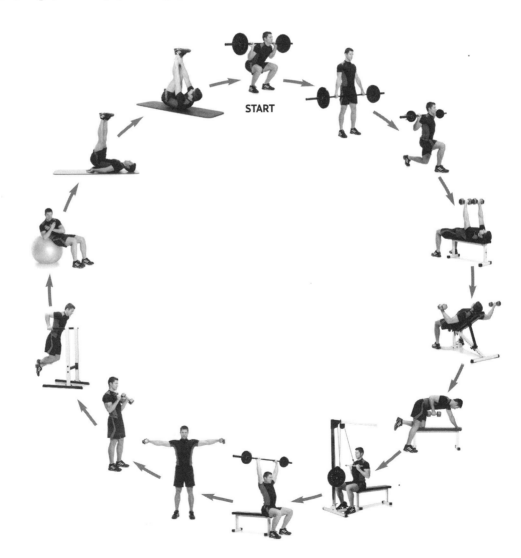

START

I Have Only 3 Days a Week

Why the Best Things Come in Threes

Just because you have enough time in your weekly schedule to do the norm doesn't mean you have to settle for average results.

Thanks to the very start of this book, you already know why the classic 3-day-a-week plan comes so highly recommended by exercise and health experts alike. Instead of repeating those benefits again, I'd like to take this time to explain one final benefit about having just 3 days: maximum muscle.

You may think that just doing what's expected when it comes to exercise—the old 3-day-a-week program means getting middle-of-the-road results. After all, if you exercise like everyone else, you're bound to look like everyone else, too, right?

Wrong!

That only happens to the exercisers who don't take advantage of what *3 whole days* can do for their body. You see, the routines in this section are still full-body programs. That means your muscles have to deal with the stress of exercise three times in one week—which is the most they can physically handle without cutting into the amount of rest they need for rebuilding. Make every workout in this section count and you'll be counting how many heads you turn after only a few weeks of sticking to these programs.

Another advantage to working your muscles on three different days is that you can challenge them in three different ways. The routines in this chapter still incorporate the basic building-block compound exercises that the 1-day-a-week and 2-day-a-week programs rely on. But with an extra day on the schedule each week, these routines can use even more of the "anytime" exercises from chapter 4. That means you'll be training your muscles with different variations of exercises for a more versatile and *more effective* workout.

The final advantage to the 3-day plan is familiarity. Because 3-day workout programs are the most popular formula used in magazines, books, and so forth, most people who exercise regularly are already used to making time for three workouts in their weekly schedules. If you're one of those people, switching your current workout to the following tried-and-true routines will be an easy adjustment guaranteed to make your muscles grow.

Here's How to Tweak Your Week

As I mentioned, nearly all the workouts in this chapter—with the exception of a few "lean-body" workouts—are full-body plans. That means, just as with the twice-a-week workouts, you need to make sure you give your muscles adequate rest so they can do their job and recover for you.

Doing the math is easy on a 3-day schedule. Most people simply exercise one day, take a rest day on the following day, and repeat twice more. (For example, they work out Monday, Wednesday, and Friday or Tuesday, Thursday, and Saturday.) Which day you decide to start doesn't really matter, as long as you follow each exercise day with a rest day and stick to exercising all 3 days. Follow that formula—and whichever of the four routines you choose, your body will never be mistaken for "average" again.

Same Time, More Results

ANGLE EVERY CHANCE YOU GET!

Using an incline or decline bench for certain chest exercises is a great way to hit your muscles from two different angles for a more thorough workout. But don't always stick with the angle you use on your first set: Changing the bench angle takes only seconds after every set, and it exhausts more muscle fibers than just one angle.

For any incline exercise bench exercise, try this twist: Instead of setting the bench at around a 45-degree angle for all your sets, try experimenting with the different angles you have at your disposal. If you have two or more sets to do, start your first set by raising the bench just one or two notches from the flat position. (This pitch will probably look like a 20- to 25-degree angle.) Then, for each remaining set, raise the bench's angle another one or two notches. Just be careful not to raise the bench too high if you're doing a lot of sets. You want to stop somewhere around a 65- to 70-degree angle—getting any closer to 90 degrees changes the exercise from a chest-building move into a shoulder-building one.)

You can try this strategy on a decline bench, too.

10 Minutes/3 Days a Week

Your Instant LEAN-BODY Plan!

All 3 Days

1 minute of low-intensity cardiovascular exercise

8 minutes of high-intensity cardio

1 minute of low-intensity cardio

Your Instant POWER Plan!

All 3 Days (Rest 45 seconds between sets)

⚡ 3 sets/**Squat** (6–8 reps)

⚡ 3 sets/**Deadlift** (6–8 reps)

⚡ 2 sets/**Bench press** (6–8 reps)

Your Instant MUSCLE Plan!

All 3 Days (Rest 30 seconds between sets)

1 set/**Squat** (8–12 reps)

1 set/**Lunge** (8–12 reps)

1 set/**Bench press** (8–12 reps)

1 set/**Bent-over row** (8–12 reps)

1 set/**Seated shoulder press** (8–12 reps)

1 set/**Biceps curl** (8–12 reps)

1 set/**Seated triceps extension** (8–12 reps)

1 set/**Crunch** (done until failure—i.e., you can't do any more)

10 Minutes/3 Days a Week

Your Instant COMPLETE-BODY Plan!

Day 1 (Rest 30 seconds between sets)

1 set/**Squat**
(8–12 reps)

1 set/**Lunge**
(8–12 reps)

1 set/**Bench press**
(8–12 reps)

1 set/**Bent-over row**
(8–12 reps)

1 set/**Seated shoulder press**
(8–12 reps)

1 set/**Biceps curl**
(8–12 reps)

1 set/**Seated triceps extension**
(8–12 reps)

1 set/**Crunch**
(done until failure)

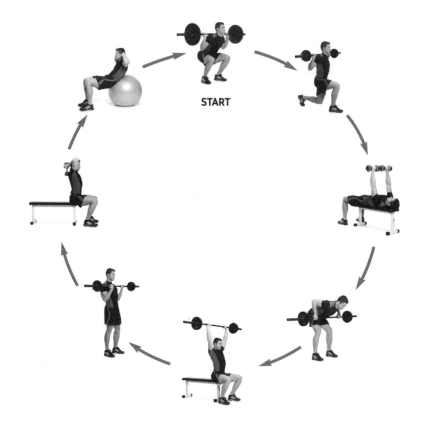

START

Day 2 (Rest 45 seconds between sets)

3 sets/**Squat**
(6–8 reps)

3 sets/**Deadlift**
(6–8 reps)

2 sets/**Bench press**
(6–8 reps)

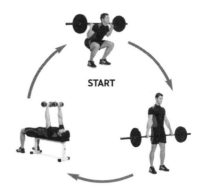

START

Day 3

1 minute of low-intensity cardiovascular exercise

8 minutes of high-intensity cardio

1 minute of low-intensity cardio

20 Minutes/3 Days a Week

Your Instant LEAN-BODY Plan!

All 3 Days

2 minutes of low-intensity cardiovascular exercise

16 minutes of medium-intensity cardio

2 minutes of low-intensity cardio

Your Instant POWER Plan!

All 3 Days (Rest 60 seconds between sets)

⚡ 4 sets/**Squat** (6–8 reps)

⚡ 3 sets/**Deadlift** (6–8 reps)

⚡ 3 sets/**Power clean** (6–8 reps)

⚡ 3 sets/**Bench press** (6–8 reps)

Your Instant MUSCLE Plan!

All 3 Days (Rest 30 seconds between sets)

3 sets/**Squat** (8–12 reps)

2 sets/**Lunge** (8–12 reps)

2 sets/**Bench press** (8–12 reps)

2 sets/**Bent-over row** (8–12 reps)

2 sets/**Seated shoulder press** (8–12 reps)

2 sets/**Biceps curl** (8–12 reps)

2 sets/**Seated triceps extension** (8–12 reps)

1 set/**Crunch** (done until failure)

1 set/**Reverse crunch** (done until failure)

20 Minutes/3 Days a Week

Your Instant **COMPLETE-BODY** Plan!

Day 1 (Rest 30 seconds between sets)

2 sets/**Squat**
(8–12 reps; 6–8 reps)

2 sets/**Deadlift**
(8–12 reps; 6–8 reps)

2 sets/**Lunge**
(8–12 reps; 6–8 reps)

2 sets/**Bench press**
(8–12 reps; 6–8 reps)

2 sets/**Bent-over row**
(8–12 reps; 6–8 reps)

2 sets/**Seated shoulder press**
(8–12 reps; 6–8 reps)

2 sets/**Biceps curl**
(8–12 reps; 6–8 reps)

2 sets/**Seated triceps extension**
(8–12 reps; 6–8 reps)

1 set/**Crunch**
(done until failure)

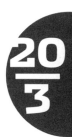

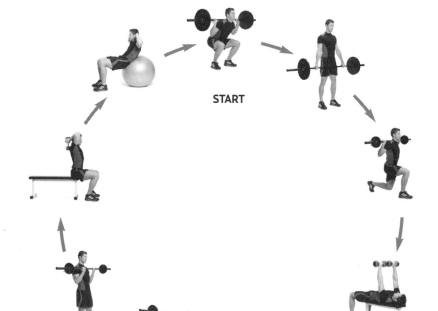

START

20 Minutes/3 Days a Week

Your Instant **COMPLETE-BODY** Plan!—cont.

Day 2 (Rest 30 seconds between sets)

2 sets/**Front squat**
(12–15 reps; 8–12 reps)

2 sets/**Deadlift**
(12–15 reps; 8–12 reps)

2 sets/**Reverse lunge**
(12–15 reps; 8–12 reps)

2 sets/**Incline press**
(12–15 reps; 8–12 reps)

2 sets/**One-arm row**
(12–15 reps; 8–12 reps)

2 sets/**Seated shoulder press**
(12–15 reps; 8–12 reps)

2 sets/**Hammer curl**
(12–15 reps; 8–12 reps)

2 sets/**Dip**
(12–15 reps; 8–12 reps)

1 set/**Reverse crunch**
(done until failure)

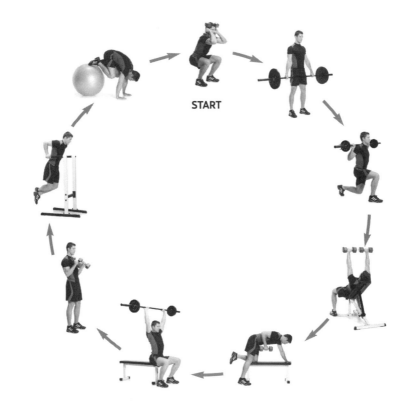

START

Day 3 (Rest 30 seconds between sets)

2 sets/**Squat**
(8–12 reps)

2 sets/**Deadlift**
(8–12 reps)

2 sets/**Lunge**
(8–12 reps)

2 sets/**Bench press**
(8–12 reps)

2 sets/**Bent-over row**
(8–12 reps)

2 sets/**Seated shoulder press**
(8–12 reps)

2 sets/**Reverse curl**
(8–12 reps)

2 sets/**Triceps pushdown**
(8–12 reps)

1 set/**V-up with a twist**
(done until failure)

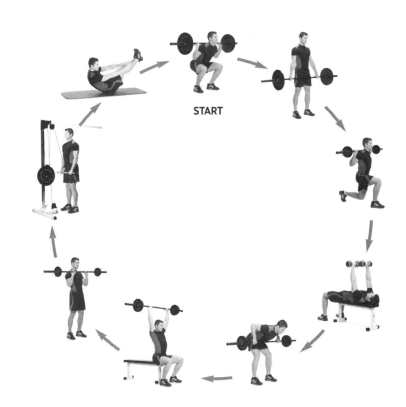

START

30 Minutes/3 Days a Week

30/3

Your Instant LEAN-BODY Plan!

All 3 Days (Rest 15 seconds between sets)

2 minutes of low-intensity cardiovascular exercise

1 set/**Squat** (12–15 reps)

1 set/**Lunge** (12–15 reps)

1 set/**Bench press** (12–15 reps)

1 set/**Bent-over row** (12–15 reps)

1 set/**Seated shoulder press** (12–15 reps)

1 set/**Biceps curl** (12–15 reps)

1 set/**Seated triceps extension** (12–15 reps)

1 set/**Crunch** (done until failure)

16 minutes of medium-intensity cardio

2 minutes of low-intensity cardio

Your Instant POWER Plan!

All 3 Days (Rest 60 seconds between sets)

⚡ 4 sets/**Squat** (6–8 reps)

⚡ 4 sets/**Deadlift** (6–8 reps)

⚡ 3 sets/**Power clean** (6–8 reps)

⚡ 3 sets/**Bench press** (6–8 reps)

⚡ 3 sets/**Push press** (6–8 reps)

⚡ 3 sets/**Bent-over row** (6–8 reps)

Your Instant MUSCLE Plan!

All 3 Days (Rest 30 seconds between sets)

4 sets/**Squat** (8–12 reps)

4 sets/**Deadlift** (8–12 reps)

3 sets/**Bench press** (8–12 reps)

3 sets/**Bent-over row** (8–12 reps)

3 sets/**Seated shoulder press** (8–12 reps)

3 sets/**Biceps curl** (8–12 reps)

3 sets/**Seated triceps extension** (8–12 reps)

1 set/**Crunch** (done until failure)

1 set/**Reverse crunch** (done until failure)

Your Instant **COMPLETE-BODY** Plan!

Day 1 (Rest 30 seconds between sets)

3 sets/**Squat**
(12–15 reps; 8–12 reps; 6–8 reps)

3 sets/**Deadlift**
(12–15 reps; 8–12 reps; 6–8 reps)

3 sets/**Lunge**
(12–15 reps; 8–12 reps; 6–8 reps)

3 sets/**Bench press**
(12–15 reps; 8–12 reps; 6–8 reps)

3 sets/**Bent-over row**
(12–15 reps; 8–12 reps; 6–8 reps)

3 sets/**Seated shoulder press**
(12–15 reps; 8–12 reps; 6–8 reps)

2 sets/**Biceps curl**
(8–12 reps; 6–8 reps)

2 sets/**Seated triceps extension**
(8–12 reps; 6–8 reps)

1 set/**Crunch**
(done until failure)

1 set/**Reverse crunch**
(done until failure)

1 set/**Side raise**
(done until failure)

30/3

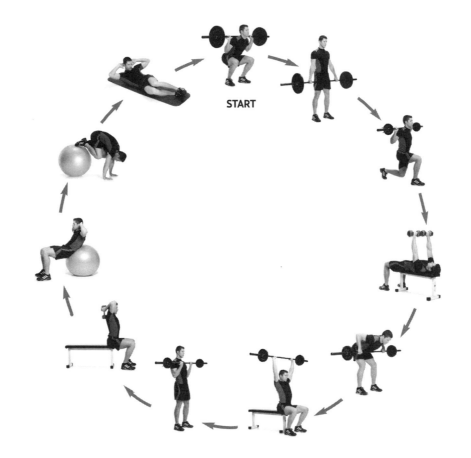

START

Your Instant **COMPLETE-BODY** Plan!—cont.

Day 2 (Rest 30 seconds between sets)

3 sets/**Front squat**
(12–15 reps; 8–12 reps; 6–8 reps)

3 sets/**Reverse lunge**
(12–15 reps; 8–12 reps; 6–8 reps)

3 sets/**Deadlift**
(12–15 reps; 8–12 reps; 6–8 reps)

3 sets/**Incline press**
(12–15 reps; 8–12 reps; 6–8 reps)

3 sets/**Lat pulldown**
(12–15 reps; 8–12 reps; 6–8 reps)

3 sets/**Push press**
(12–15 reps; 8–12 reps; 6–8 reps)

2 sets/**Hammer curl**
(8–12 reps; 6–8 reps)

2 sets/**Triceps pushdown**
(8–12 reps; 6–8 reps)

1 set/**Twisting crunch**
(done until failure)

1 set/**Twisting toe touch**
(done until failure)

1 set/**V-up with a twist**
(done until failure)

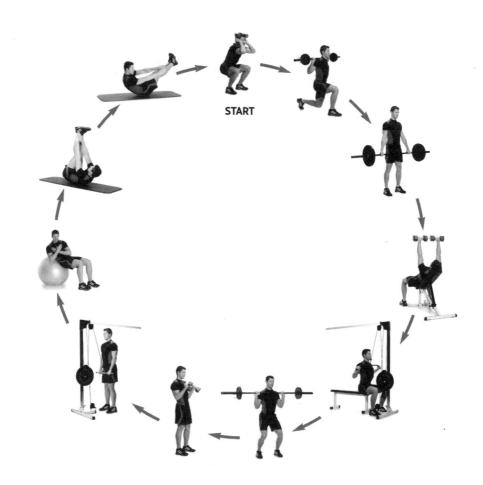

START

Day 3 (Rest 30 seconds between sets)

3 sets/**Power clean**
(12–15 reps; 8–12 reps; 6–8 reps)

3 sets/**Side lunge**
(12–15 reps; 8–12 reps; 6–8 reps)

3 sets/**Decline press**
(12–15 reps; 8–12 reps; 6–8 reps)

3 sets/**Close-grip pulldown**
(12–15 reps; 8–12 reps; 6–8 reps)

3 sets/**Push press**
(12–15 reps; 8–12 reps; 6–8 reps)

3 sets/**Front raise**
(12–15 reps; 8–12 reps; 6–8 reps)

2 sets/**Reverse curl**
(8–12 reps; 6–8 reps)

2 sets/**Dip**
(8–12 reps; 6–8 reps)

1 set/**Crunch**
(done until failure)

1 set/**Reverse crunch**
(done until failure)

1 set/**V-up with a twist**
(done until failure)

30/3

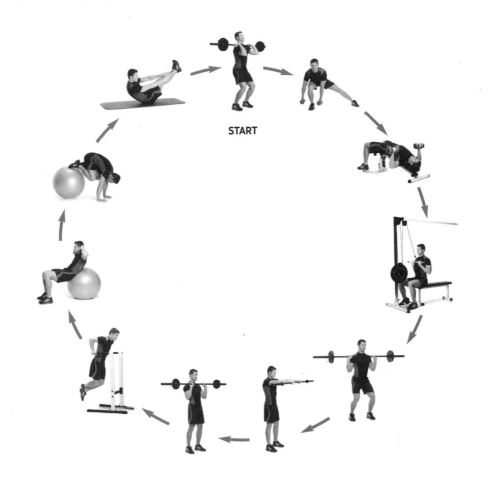

START

45 Minutes/3 Days a Week

Your Instant LEAN-BODY Plan!

Days 1 + 3 (Rest 15 seconds between sets)

2 minutes of low-intensity cardiovascular exercise
2 sets/**Squat** (12–15 reps)
2 sets/**Lunge** (12–15 reps)
2 sets/**Bench press** (12–15 reps)
2 sets/**One-arm row** (12–15 reps)
2 sets/**Seated shoulder press** (12–15 reps)
2 sets/**Biceps curl** (12–15 reps)
2 sets/**Seated triceps extension** (12–15 reps)
1 set/**Crunch** (done until failure)
1 set/**Reverse crunch** (done until failure)
20 minutes of medium-intensity cardio
3 minutes of low-intensity cardio

Day 2 (Rest 15 seconds between sets)

2 minutes of low-intensity cardiovascular exercise
1 set/**Squat** (12–15 reps)
1 set/**Lunge** (12–15 reps)
1 set/**Bench press** (12–15 reps)
1 set/**One-arm row** (12–15 reps)
1 set/**Seated shoulder press** (12–15 reps)
1 set/**Biceps curl** (12–15 reps)
1 set/**Seated triceps extension** (12–15 reps)
1 set/**Crunch** (done until failure)
1 set/**Reverse crunch** (done until failure)
30 minutes of medium-intensity cardio
2 minutes of low-intensity cardio

Your Instant POWER Plan!

Days 1 + 3 (Rest 90 seconds between sets)

5 sets/**Squat** (6–8 reps)
4 sets/**Deadlift** (6–8 reps)
4 sets/**Bench press** (6–8 reps)
3 sets/**Push press** (6–8 reps)
3 sets/**Bent-over row** (6–8 reps)
2 sets/**Biceps curl** (6–8 reps)
2 sets/**Dip** (6–8 reps)

Day 2 (Rest 90 seconds between sets)

5 sets/**Squat** (6–8 reps)
4 sets/**Power clean** (6–8 reps)
4 sets/**Incline press** (6–8 reps)
3 sets/**Seated shoulder press** (6–8 reps)
2 sets/**One-arm row** (6–8 reps)
2 sets/**Biceps curl** (6–8 reps)
2 sets/**Dip** (6–8 reps)

Your Instant MUSCLE Plan!

Day 1 (Rest 60 seconds between sets)

4 sets/**Squat** (8–12 reps)

4 sets/**Deadlift** (8–12 reps)

4 sets/**Bench press** (8–12 reps)

4 sets/**Incline press** (8–12 reps)

3 sets/**Bent-over row** (8–12 reps)

3 sets/**Pullover** (8–12 reps)

3 sets/**Seated shoulder press** (8–12 reps)

3 sets/**Lateral raise** (8–12 reps)

3 sets/**Biceps curl** (8–12 reps)

3 sets/**Seated triceps extension** (8–12 reps)

1 set/**Reverse crunch** (done until failure)

1 set/**Twisting crunch** (done until failure)

Day 2 (Rest 60 seconds between sets)

4 sets/**Front squat** (8–12 reps)

3 sets/**Lunge** (8–12 reps)

4 sets/**Bench press** (8–12 reps)

3 sets/**Chest fly** (8–12 reps)

3 sets/**Lat pulldown** (8–12 reps)

3 sets/**Close-grip pulldown** (8–12 reps)

3 sets/**Seated shoulder press** (8–12 reps)

3 sets/**Bent-over reverse raise** (8–12 reps)

3 sets/**Hammer curl** (8–12 reps)

3 sets/**Dip** (8–12 reps)

1 set/**Crunch** (done until failure)

1 set/**Twisting leg thrust** (done until failure)

Day 3 (Rest 60 seconds between sets)

4 sets/**Squat** (8–12 reps)

4 sets/**Deadlift** (8–12 reps)

4 sets/**Bench press** (8–12 reps)

3 sets/**Decline press** (8–12 reps)

2 sets/**One-arm row** (8–12 reps)

3 sets/**Upright row** (8–12 reps)

3 sets/**Seated shoulder press** (8–12 reps)

3 sets/**Shrug** (8–12 reps)

3 sets/**Reverse curl** (8–12 reps)

3 sets/**Triceps pushdown** (8–12 reps)

1 set/**Side raise** (done until failure)

1 set/**V-up with a twist** (done until failure)

60/3

60 Minutes/3 Days a Week

Your Instant **COMPLETE-BODY** Plan!

Days 1 + 3 (Rest 60 seconds between sets)

4 sets/**Squat**
(12–15 reps; 8–12 reps; 6–8 reps; 6–8 reps)

4 sets/**Deadlift**
(12–15 reps; 8–12 reps; 6–8 reps; 6–8 reps)

3 sets/**Lunge**
(12–15 reps; 8–12 reps; 6–8 reps)

3 sets/**Bench press**
(12–15 reps; 8–12 reps; 6–8 reps)

3 sets/**Incline press**
(12–15 reps; 8–12 reps; 6–8 reps)

3 sets/**Bent-over row**
(12–15 reps; 8–12 reps; 6–8 reps)

3 sets/**Lat pulldown**
(12–15 reps; 8–12 reps; 6–8 reps)

3 sets/**Seated shoulder press**
(12–15 reps; 8–12 reps; 6–8 reps)

3 sets/**Lateral raise**
(12–15 reps; 8–12 reps; 6–8 reps)

2 sets/**Biceps curl**
(8–12 reps; 6–8 reps)

2 sets/**Seated triceps extension**
(8–12 reps; 6–8 reps)

1 set/**Crunch**
(done until failure)

1 set/**Reverse crunch**
(done until failure)

1 set/**V-up with a twist**
(done until failure)

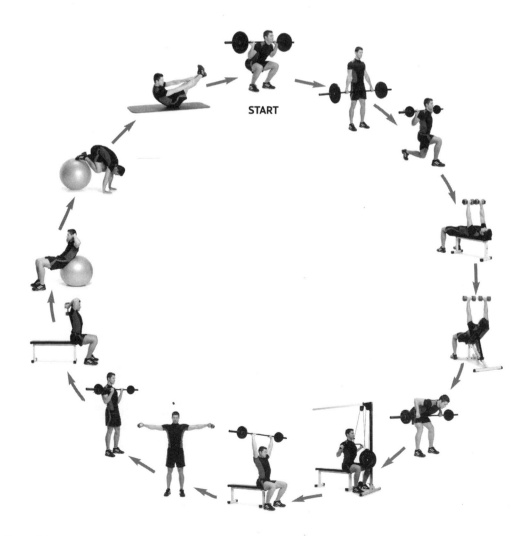

START

Day 2 (Rest 60 seconds between sets)

4 sets/**Reverse lunge**
(12–15 reps; 8–12 reps; 6–8 reps; 6–8 reps)

4 sets/**Bench press**
(12–15 reps; 8–12 reps; 6–8 reps; 6–8 reps)

3 sets/**Incline fly**
(12–15 reps; 8–12 reps; 6–8 reps)

3 sets/**One-arm row**
(12–15 reps; 8–12 reps; 6–8 reps)

3 sets/**Close-grip pulldown**
(12–15 reps; 8–12 reps; 6–8 reps)

3 sets/**Seated shoulder press**
(12–15 reps; 8–12 reps; 6–8 reps)

3 sets/**Lateral raise**
(12–15 reps; 8–12 reps; 6–8 reps)

2 sets/**Hammer curl**
(8–12 reps; 6–8 reps)

2 sets/**Dip**
(8–12 reps; 6–8 reps)

1 set/**Twisting crunch**
(done until failure)

1 set/**Twisting leg thrust**
(done until failure)

1 set/**Twisting toe touch**
(done until failure)

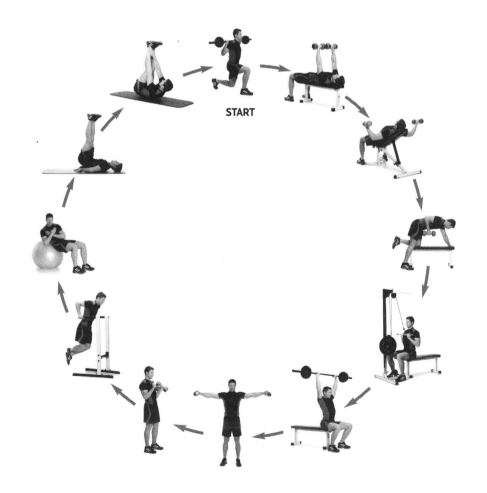

START

I Have 4 Days a Week

The 4-Day Payoff

Adding an extra day to the average exercise plan can mean you've crossed the border from amateur to advanced, especially if you plan on spending those 4 days working out for 30 minutes a day or more. Is that you? Are you ready to step your workouts up a notch? That's good, because I'm about to show you just how easy it can be.

It's time for a quick math lesson, so blow the dust off your abacus. If you're supposed to rest your muscles at least 48 hours between workouts, then isn't trying to train 4 days a week impossible?

Not necessarily.

It *is* impossible . . . if you stick strictly to the full-body routines I've prescribed in the 1-, 2-, and 3-day-a-week sections. But if you're planning on putting in 4 days this week, then your "training every muscle group on the same day" sessions are over. You now get to take advantage of an intermediate style of workout known as a *split routine.*

Instead of hitting all your muscles on one day, you're now going to be splitting your full-body

workout into two separate workouts—training half of your body on one day and the other half on the next day. Dividing your workouts in this way lets you train your muscles with more intensity for even better results than you're used to.

How does it do that? Simple!

Breaking your workout up into two parts gives you twice the amount of time to spend on the muscles in each workout. That means you can do twice as many exercises—on average—per muscle group, which works them more thoroughly by incorporating additional muscle fibers as you exercise.

Being able to add even more of the "anytime" exercises means you'll also be able to give your larger muscle groups the full attention they need in order to really transform for you. As you know from your earlier reading in this book, many of your larger muscles are divided into several different sections. For example, your shoulders are made up of three muscles: your anterior, medial, and posterior heads. Even though the basic, compound exercises used in the earlier programs in this book—the shoulder press, for example—are perfect for working the front and side parts of your shoulders, it leaves out the back of your shoulders. Splitting your routine—thanks to having 4 days to do so—means you'll be able to add other exercises to isolate parts of your larger muscles that the basic programs may miss.

Even your smaller muscles can benefit from having more exercises to choose from, since they are usually the last areas you focus on when you're time-deprived. For example, your calves—which are made up of two separate muscles: the gastrocnemius and the soleus—require different types of exercises to get them to develop fully. The gastrocnemius—the upper and outer part of your calves—is activated when you do exercises from a standing position, whereas the soleus—which lies under-neath—is best worked when doing exercises from a seated position. Splitting your routine finally gives you enough time to try both types of exercises—a time trick that other smaller muscles, such as your biceps and triceps, can also benefit from.

Here's How to Tweak Your Week

Unlike your 1-, 2-, or 3-day routines, these 4-day routines require you to exercise 2 days in a row without taking a day off in between. But don't worry. These routines are already organized to ensure that you'll never train the same muscle group 2 days in a row.

TIME TWEAKS!

Spend More Time . . . Taking Things Slow!

When time isn't an issue, try lifting your weights at a slower pace. This technique—known as the "super slow" method—is a weight-lifting trick that's simple to do. Instead of lifting weights with a 2-seconds-up, 2-seconds-down pace, you'll switch to a lighter weight and spend exactly 6 to 10 seconds lifting the weight and 6 to 10 seconds lowering it. One set will end up taking you around 2½ to 3 minutes to finish, but trying this tweak every once in a while can be worth the extra time you put into it.

You'll focus harder. The slower you perform an exercise, the less risk you have of creating a sense of momentum. Slowing it down to this extreme makes it virtually impossible for you to lift the weight with anything except the muscles you're trying to shape and improve. That's why most exercisers notice results from this technique in as little as 2 weeks.

You'll feel better. Using the "super slow" technique is also a lot safer for the injury-prone, since many exercise strains and pains occur within smaller stabilizing muscles that become overworked when you're handling heavier loads of weight. If you're worried that exercising with lighter weights won't build strength in your muscles as effectively, don't be! Using less weight at a slower tempo achieves the same results as heavier weights when it comes to improving the strength of muscles—without adding any undue size for those not looking to get too big.

You'll finish faster. Spending two to three times longer doing an exercise makes this technique seem like a time waster, but it's actually a time saver. One set of 15 repetitions performed at an average tempo takes about a minute and a half to finish, with a 30- to 45-second period of rest between sets. Add it up, and you'll find that doing a total of 3 sets per exercise at the regular pace can make one move take more than 6 minutes to finish! On the other hand, 1 set of 15 repetitions done at a super-slow pace may take up to 3 minutes, but that's all you'll need to do. One set of an exercise in slow motion can work muscles just as hard as 3 regular sets, while placing less stress on joints and tendons. Add a minute of rest and 1 set only takes 4 minutes to complete, shaving your workout time by 33 percent.

TIME TWEAKS!

Spend More Time . . . Focusing On the Muscles You Can't See!

It's easy to concentrate on the muscles you can see in the mirror as you train them. But focusing on the ones you can't see—your trapezius, rear shoulders, upper and lower back, gluteals, hamstrings, and calves—is a lot harder to remember. It's worth the effort, though: Making a "mind-muscle" connection with these unsung, unseen heroes of your physique can produce faster results. These three tricks will help you do just that.

Make yourself imagine. Shutting your lids as you lift helps you tune in to which muscles are doing the job of raising the weight, as well as keeping out distractions. This method shouldn't be used for every exercise—especially not for standing exercises that require you to stay balanced—but it's ideal for pulldown exercises (for your upper back), one-arm rows, and lying leg exercises.

Make a friend. Let a training partner lightly touch the muscles you're working as you exercise—it can help you figure out whether you're using them completely or cheating with other surrounding muscles. This technique works perfectly for all back and leg exercises, as well as for your abs—since you should never look down as you train them.

Make a muscle. Flexing your muscles may seem a bit ostentatious, but it stresses your muscle fibers even more, so you can feel them after each set. Once you finish a set, try tightening the muscles you've just trained for 4 to 5 seconds.

You'll work your chest, shoulders, triceps, and abdominals on the first day, and your legs, back, biceps, and abdominals on the second day. To be honest, there are several ways you can split up your routine, but because this book is all about making the wisest and most convenient decisions when it comes to exercise, your routines are divided so that muscle groups that typically work together will stay together!

You see, whenever you do an exercise for your chest, you indirectly work your shoulder and triceps muscles, because they also help lift the weight. The same partnership takes place between your back and your biceps. Whenever you do an exercise to strengthen or shape your back, your biceps—and even your forearms—also get a workout, whether they want one or not.

If you train your chest on one day and your shoulders and triceps the next, your shoulders and triceps never get a full 48 hours to rest, since they are indirectly worked the day before. What this does is leave these muscles weaker over time, which not only prevents *them* from seeing results

but also prevents your chest from seeing as many either, since they are left too weak to help out. Arranging your muscles wisely by pairing them up in the right combinations will let you exhaust them more thoroughly, and it'll also let them rest the next day, when you're training other muscles that don't involve them as much or at all.

You may notice that in most of these routines, you'll still work your abdominal muscles with every workout. That's because your abs are slightly more capable of handling the stress of exercise on an everyday basis. However, to help guarantee that your abs get a rest, these routines divide up the types of exercises to work different sections of your rectus abdominis—either the upper or lower portions—on different days.

Here's the smartest plan for a 4-day schedule: Start your week with Day 1, do Day 2 the very next day, then take a day off. Then repeat the cycle again. This gives your individual muscles at least 48 hours of rest between training days. Now that you're ready to cut your workouts in half, use these routines to achieve your goals twice as fast!

10 Minutes/4 Days a Week

Your Instant LEAN-BODY Plan!

All 4 Days

1 minute of low-intensity cardiovascular exercise

8 minutes of high-intensity cardio

1 minute of low-intensity cardio

Your Instant POWER Plan!

Days 1 + 3 (Rest 45 seconds between sets)

- 2 sets/**Power clean** (6–8 reps)
- 2 sets/**Bench press** (6–8 reps)
- 2 sets/**Push press** (6–8 reps)
- 2 sets/**Dip** (6–8 reps)

Days 2 + 4 (Rest 45 seconds between sets)

- 3 sets/**Squat** (6–8 reps)
- 3 sets/**Deadlift** (6–8 reps)
- 2 sets/**Bent-over row** (6–8 reps)

Your Instant MUSCLE Plan!

Days 1 + 3 (Rest 30 seconds between sets)

3 sets/**Bench press** (8–12 reps)

2 sets/**Seated shoulder press** (8–12 reps)

2 sets/**Seated triceps extension** (8–12 reps)

1 set/**Crunch** (done until failure—i.e., you can't do any more)

Days 2 + 4 (Rest 30 seconds between sets)

3 sets/**Squat** (8–12 reps)

2 sets/**Bent-over row** (8–12 reps)

2 sets/**Biceps curl** (8–12 reps)

1 set/**Reverse crunch** (done until failure)

10 Minutes/4 Days a Week

Your Instant COMPLETE-BODY Plan!

Day 1 (Rest 30 seconds between sets)

2 sets/**Bench press**
(8–12 reps)

2 sets/**Seated shoulder press**
(8–12 reps)

2 sets/**Seated triceps extension**
(8–12 reps)

2 sets/**Crunch**
(each set done until failure)

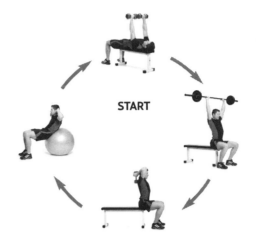

Day 2 (Rest 30 seconds between sets)

2 sets/**Squat**
(8–12 reps)

2 sets/**Lunge**
(8–12 reps)

2 sets/**Bent-over row**
(8–12 reps)

2 sets/**Biceps curl**
(8–12 reps)

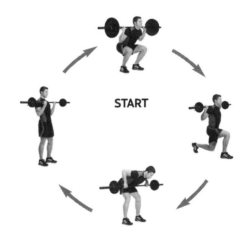

Your Instant COMPLETE-BODY Plan!—cont.

Day 3 (Rest 15 seconds between sets)

2 sets/**Incline press**
(12–15 reps)

2 sets/**Lateral raise**
(12–15 reps)

2 sets/**Triceps pushdown**
(12–15 reps)

2 sets/**Reverse crunch**
(each set done until failure)

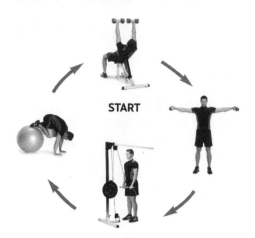

START

Day 4 (Rest 15 seconds between sets)

2 sets/**Front squat**
(12–15 reps)

2 sets/**Reverse lunge**
(12–15 reps)

2 sets/**Lat pulldown**
(12–15 reps)

2 sets/**Hammer curl**
(12–15 reps)

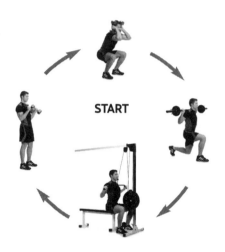

START

20 Minutes/4 Days a Week

Your Instant LEAN-BODY Plan!

All 4 Days

2 minutes of low-intensity cardiovascular exercise

16 minutes of medium-intensity cardio

2 minutes of low-intensity cardio

Your Instant POWER Plan!

Days 1 + 3 (Rest 60 seconds between sets)

- 4 sets/**Power clean** (6–8 reps)
- 3 sets/**Bench press** (6–8 reps)
- 3 sets/**Push press** (6–8 reps)
- 3 sets/**Dip** (6–8 reps)

Days 2 + 4 (Rest 60 seconds between sets)

- 4 sets/**Squat** (6–8 reps)
- 4 sets/**Deadlift** (6–8 reps)
- 3 sets/**Bent-over row** (6–8 reps)
- 2 sets/**Biceps curl** (6–8 reps)

Your Instant MUSCLE Plan!

Days 1 + 3 (Rest 30 seconds between sets)

- 3 sets/**Bench press** (8–12 reps)
- 2 sets/**Incline press** (8–12 reps)
- 3 sets/**Seated shoulder press** (8–12 reps)
- 2 sets/**Lateral raise** (8–12 reps)
- 3 sets/**Seated triceps extension** (8–12 reps)
- 2 sets/**Triceps pushdown** (8–12 reps)
- 1 set/**Crunch** (done until failure)
- 1 set/**Reverse crunch** (done until failure)

Days 2 + 4 (Rest 30 seconds between sets)

- 3 sets/**Squat** (8–12 reps)
- 3 sets/**Lunge** (8–12 reps)
- 3 sets/**Bent-over row** (8–12 reps)
- 2 sets/**Lat pulldown** (8–12 reps)
- 2 sets/**Biceps curl** (8–12 reps)
- 2 sets/**Reverse curl** (8–12 reps)
- 1 set/**Crunch** (done until failure)
- 1 set/**Reverse crunch** (done until failure)

20/4

20 Minutes/4 Days a Week

Your Instant COMPLETE-BODY Plan!

Day 1 (Rest 30 seconds between sets)

3 sets/**Bench press**
(12–15 reps; 8–12 reps; 6–8 reps)

2 sets/**Incline press**
(8–12 reps; 6–8 reps)

3 sets/**Seated shoulder press**
(12–15 reps; 8–12 reps; 6–8 reps)

2 sets/**Lateral raise**
(8–12 reps; 6–8 reps)

3 sets/**Seated triceps extension**
(12–15 reps; 8–12 reps; 6–8 reps)

2 sets/**Triceps pushdown**
(8–12 reps; 6–8 reps)

1 set/**Crunch**
(done until failure)

1 set/**Reverse crunch**
(done until failure)

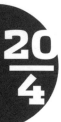

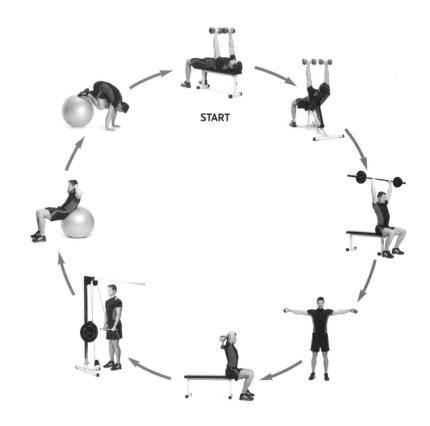

START

Day 2 (Rest 30 seconds between sets)

3 sets/**Squat**
(12–15 reps; 8–12 reps; 6–8 reps)

3 sets/**Lunge**
(12–15 reps; 8–12 reps; 6–8 reps)

3 sets/**Bent-over row**
(12–15 reps; 8–12 reps; 6–8 reps)

2 sets/**Lat pulldown**
(8–12 reps; 6–8 reps)

2 sets/**Biceps curl**
(8–12 reps; 6–8 reps)

2 sets/**Reverse curl**
(8–12 reps; 6–8 reps)

1 set/**Side raise**
(done until failure)

1 set/**V-up with a twist**
(done until failure)

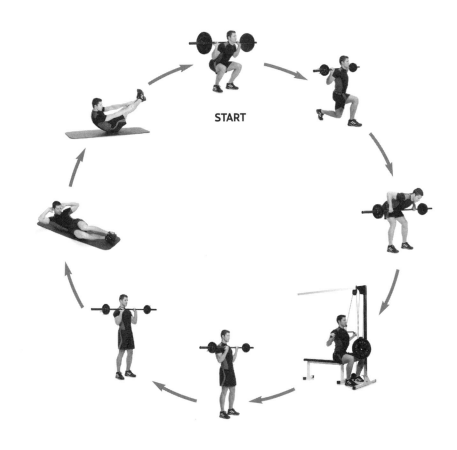

START

20
4

Your Instant **COMPLETE-BODY** Plan!—cont.

Day 3 (Rest 30 seconds between sets)

3 sets/**Bench press**
(12–15 reps; 8–12 reps; 6–8 reps)

2 sets/**Chest fly**
(8–12 reps; 6–8 reps)

3 sets/**Seated shoulder press**
(12–15 reps; 8–12 reps; 6–8 reps)

2 sets/**Bent-over reverse raise**
(8–12 reps; 6–8 reps)

3 sets/**Triceps pushdown**
(12–15 reps; 8–12 reps; 6–8 reps)

2 sets/**Dip**
(8–12 reps; 6–8 reps)

1 set/**Crunch**
(done until failure)

1 set/**Reverse crunch**
(done until failure)

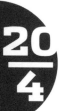

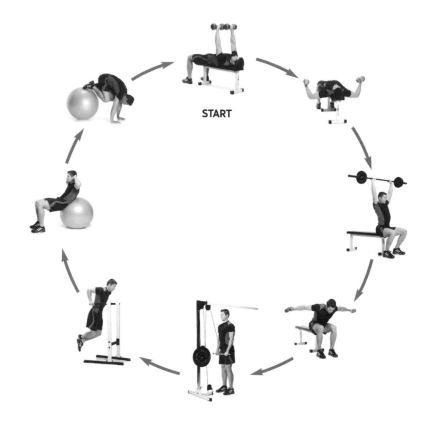

START

Day 4 (Rest 30 seconds between sets)

3 sets/**Front squat**
(12–15 reps; 8–12 reps; 6–8 reps)

3 sets/**Reverse lunge**
(12–15 reps; 8–12 reps; 6–8 reps)

2 sets/**One-arm row**
(8–12 reps; 6–8 reps)

2 sets/**Close-grip pulldown**
(8–12 reps; 6–8 reps)

2 sets/**Hammer curl**
(8–12 reps; 6–8 reps)

2 sets/**Preacher curl**
(8–12 reps; 6–8 reps)

1 set/**Side raise**
(done until failure)

1 set/**V-up with a twist**
(done until failure)

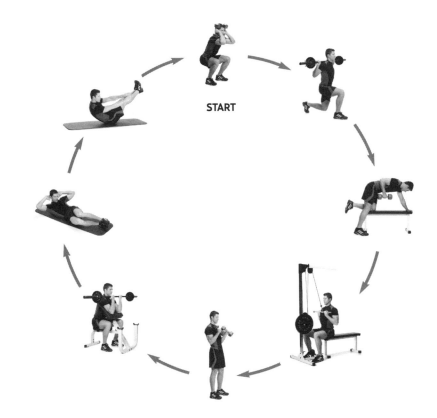

START

20
4

30 Minutes/4 Days a Week

Your Instant LEAN-BODY Plan!

Days 1 + 3 (Rest 15 seconds between sets)

2 minutes of low-intensity cardiovascular exercise

2 sets/**Bench press** (12–15 reps)

2 sets/**Seated shoulder press** (12–15 reps)

2 sets/**Seated triceps extension** (12–15 reps)

2 sets/**Crunch** (each set done until failure)

16 minutes of medium-intensity cardio

2 minutes of low-intensity cardio

Days 2 + 4 (Rest 15 seconds between sets)

2 minutes of low-intensity cardiovascular exercise

2 sets/**Squat** (12–15 reps)

2 sets/**Lunge** (12–15 reps)

2 sets/**Bent-over row** (12–15 reps)

2 sets/**Biceps curl** (12–15 reps)

16 minutes of medium-intensity cardio

2 minutes of low-intensity cardio

Your Instant POWER Plan!

Days 1 + 3 (Rest 90 seconds between sets)

⚡ 3 sets/**Bench press** (6–8 reps)

⚡ 3 sets/**Incline press** (6–8 reps)

⚡ 3 sets/**Decline press** (6–8 reps)

⚡ 3 sets/**Seated shoulder press** (6–8 reps)

⚡ 3 sets/**Dip** (6–8 reps)

Days 2 + 4 (Rest 90 seconds between sets)

⚡ 4 sets/**Squat** (6–8 reps)

⚡ 4 sets/**Deadlift** (6–8 reps)

⚡ 3 sets/**Lunge** (6–8 reps)

⚡ 2 sets/**Bent-over row** (6–8 reps)

⚡ 2 sets/**Biceps curl** (6–8 reps)

Your Instant MUSCLE Plan!

Days 1 + 3 (Rest 30 seconds between sets)

4 sets/**Bench press** (8–12 reps)

3 sets/**Incline press** (8–12 reps)

2 sets/**Chest fly** (8–12 reps)

3 sets/**Seated shoulder press** (8–12 reps)

3 sets/**Lateral raise** (8–12 reps)

2 sets/**Bent-over reverse raise** (8–12 reps)

3 sets/**Seated triceps extension** (8–12 reps)

3 sets/**Triceps pushdown** (8–12 reps)

1 set/**Crunch** (done until failure)

1 set/**Reverse crunch** (done until failure)

Days 2 + 4 (Rest 30 seconds between sets)

4 sets/**Squat** (8–12 reps)

3 sets/**Deadlift** (8–12 reps)

3 sets/**Lunge** (8–12 reps)

3 sets/**One-arm row** (8–12 reps)

3 sets/**Biceps curl** (8–12 reps)

3 sets/**Reverse curl** (8–12 reps)

3 sets/**Standing calf raise** (8–12 reps)

1 set/**Side raise** (done until failure)

1 set/**V-up with a twist** (done until failure)

30/4

TIME TWEAKS!

Some Rules to Remember Before You Try the "Super Slow" Technique

☒ When you're working out super slow, always go with at least a 40 to 50 percent lighter weight than you'd usually use. For example, if you normally grab 30-pound dumbbells for a specific exercise, grab 15-pound dumbbells for the slow version.

☒ Think notes instead of numbers. You may not be going as slow as you think: It should take you at least 6 seconds to raise the weight and 6 seconds to lower it, but it's easy to count fast to rush through an exercise. Instead, try this trick. Before you exercise, think of a song verse that you know by heart, then sing it in your head while watching the clock to see which words fall at the

6- and 12-second marks. Then, as you lift, repeat that song in your head to ensure you're keeping the right pace every time.

☒ Do 1 set—or 2, if you feel up to it—per exercise. Going over that number may feel like it will yield more results, but it only makes it more difficult for your body to recover.

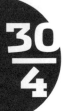

30 Minutes/4 Days a Week

Your Instant COMPLETE-BODY Plan!

Day 1 (Rest 30 seconds between sets)

4 sets/**Bench press**
(12–15 reps; 8–12 reps; 6–8 reps; 6–8 reps)

3 sets/**Incline fly**
(12–15 reps; 8–12 reps; 6–8 reps)

3 sets/**Decline press**
(12–15 reps; 8–12 reps; 6–8 reps)

3 sets/**Seated shoulder press**
(12–15 reps; 8–12 reps; 6–8 reps)

3 sets/**Lateral raise**
(12–15 reps; 8–12 reps; 6–8 reps)

3 sets/**Seated triceps extension**
(12–15 reps; 8–12 reps; 6–8 reps)

3 sets/**Triceps pushdown**
(12–15 reps; 8–12 reps; 6–8 reps)

1 set/**Crunch**
(done until failure)

1 set/**Reverse crunch**
(done until failure)

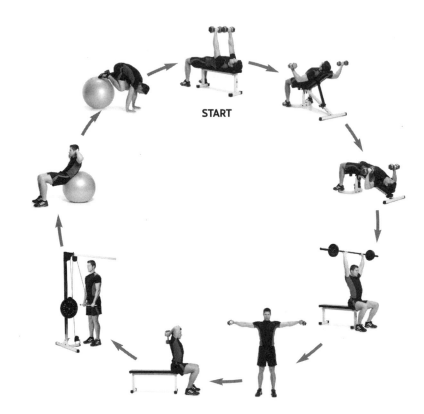

START

Day 2 (Rest 30 seconds between sets)

3 sets/**Squat**
(12–15 reps; 8–12 reps; 6–8 reps)

3 sets/**Lunge**
(12–15 reps; 8–12 reps; 6–8 reps)

2 sets/**Side lunge**
(12–15 reps; 8–12 reps)

3 sets/**Bent-over row**
(12–15 reps; 8–12 reps; 6–8 reps)

3 sets/**Lat pulldown**
(8–12 reps; 8–12 reps; 6–8 reps)

3 sets/**Biceps curl**
(8–12 reps; 8–12 reps; 6–8 reps)

3 sets/**Reverse curl**
(8–12 reps; 8–12 reps; 6–8 reps)

2 sets/**Standing calf raise**
(12–15 reps; 8–12 reps)

1 set/**Side raise**
(done until failure)

1 set/**V-up with a twist**
(done until failure)

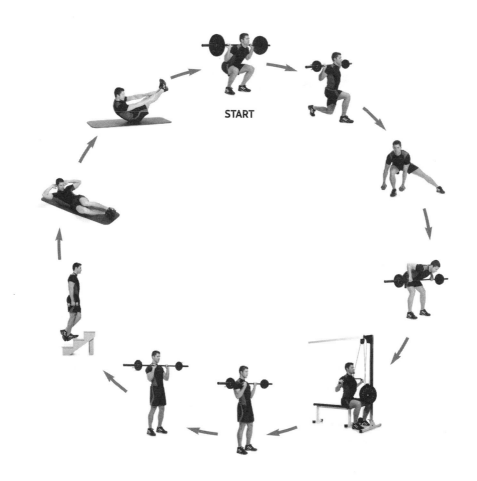

START

Your Instant **COMPLETE-BODY** Plan!—cont.

Day 3 (Rest 30 seconds between sets)

4 sets/**Bench press**
(12–15 reps; 8–12 reps; 6–8 reps; 6–8 reps)

3 sets/**Chest fly**
(12–15 reps; 8–12 reps; 6–8 reps)

3 sets/**Seated shoulder press**
(12–15 reps; 8–12 reps; 6–8 reps)

3 sets/**Front raise**
(12–15 reps; 8–12 reps; 6–8 reps)

3 sets/**Bent-over reverse raise**
(12–15 reps; 8–12 reps; 6–8 reps)

3 sets/**Lying triceps press**
(12–15 reps; 8–12 reps; 6–8 reps)

2 sets/**One-arm triceps extension**
(12–15 reps; 8–12 reps)

1 set/**Crunch**
(done until failure)

1 set/**Reverse crunch**
(done until failure)

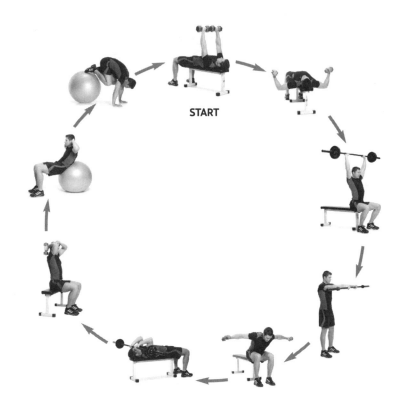

START

Day 4 (Rest 30 seconds between sets)

3 sets/**Front squat**
(12–15 reps; 8–12 reps; 6–8 reps)

3 sets/**Reverse lunge**
(12–15 reps; 8–12 reps; 6–8 reps)

3 sets/**One-arm row**
(12–15 reps; 8–12 reps; 6–8 reps)

3 sets/**Close-grip pulldown**
(8–12 reps; 8–12 reps; 6–8 reps)

3 sets/**Hammer curl**
(8–12 reps; 8–12 reps; 6–8 reps)

2 sets/**Preacher curl**
(8–12 reps; 6–8 reps)

1 set/**Wrist curl**
(8–12 reps)

1 set/**Wrist extension**
(8–12 reps)

2 sets/**Seated calf raise**
(12–15 reps; 8–12 reps)

1 set/**Side raise**
(done until failure)

1 set/**V-up with a twist**
(done until failure)

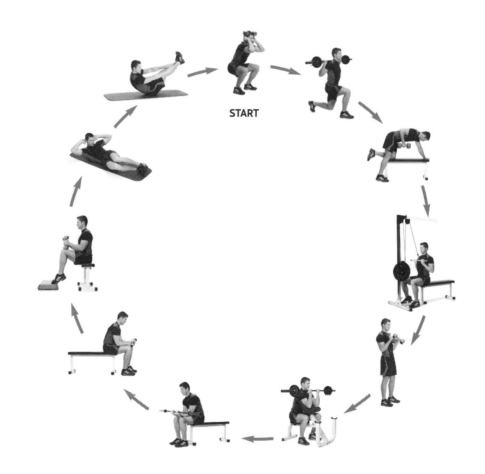

START

45 Minutes/4 Days a Week

Your Instant LEAN-BODY Plan!

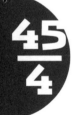

Days 1 + 3 (Rest 15 seconds between sets)

2 minutes of low-intensity cardiovascular exercise

2 sets/**Bench press** (12–15 reps)

2 sets/**Chest fly** (12–15 reps)

2 sets/**Seated shoulder press** (12–15 reps)

2 sets/**Lateral raise** (12–15 reps)

2 sets/**Seated triceps extension** (12–15 reps)

2 sets/**Kickback** (12–15 reps)

2 sets/**Crunch** (each set done until failure)

2 sets/**Reverse crunch** (each set done until failure)

20 minutes of medium-intensity cardio

3 minutes of low-intensity cardio

Days 2 + 4 (Rest 15 seconds between sets)

2 minutes of low-intensity cardiovascular exercise

3 sets/**Squat** (12–15 reps)

3 sets/**Lunge** (12–15 reps)

2 sets/**Bent-over row** (12–15 reps)

2 sets/**Lat pulldown** (12–15 reps)

2 sets/**Biceps curl** (12–15 reps)

2 sets/**Crunch** (each set done until failure)

2 sets/**Reverse crunch** (each set done until failure)

20 minutes of medium-intensity cardio

3 minutes of low-intensity cardio

Your Instant POWER Plan!

Days 1 + 3 (Rest 90 seconds between sets)

- ⚡ 4 sets/**Bench press** (6–8 reps)
- ⚡ 3 sets/**Incline press** (6–8 reps)
- ⚡ 3 sets/**Decline press** (6–8 reps)
- ⚡ 4 sets/**Seated shoulder press** (6–8 reps)
- ⚡ 4 sets/**Dip** (6–8 reps)
- ⚡ 3 sets/**Triceps pushdown** (6–8 reps)
- ⚡ 1 set/**Crunch** (done until failure)
- ⚡ 1 set/**Reverse crunch** (done until failure)

Days 2 + 4 (Rest 90 seconds between sets)

- ⚡ 5 sets/**Squat** (6–8 reps)
- ⚡ 5 sets/**Deadlift** (6–8 reps)
- ⚡ 3 sets/**Lunge** (6–8 reps)
- ⚡ 3 sets/**Bent-over row** (6–8 reps)
- ⚡ 3 sets/**Lat pulldown** (6–8 reps)
- ⚡ 2 sets/**Biceps curl** (6–8 reps)
- ⚡ 1 set/**Crunch** (done until failure)
- ⚡ 1 set/**Reverse crunch** (done until failure)

Your Instant MUSCLE Plan!

Days 1 + 3 (Rest 45 seconds between sets)

- 4 sets/**Bench press** (8–12 reps)
- 4 sets/**Incline press** (8–12 reps)
- 3 sets/**Decline press** (8–12 reps)
- 4 sets/**Seated shoulder press** (8–12 reps)
- 3 sets/**Lateral raise** (8–12 reps)
- 3 sets/**Bent-over reverse raise** (8–12 reps)
- 3 sets/**Seated triceps extension** (8–12 reps)
- 3 sets/**Triceps pushdown** (8–12 reps)
- 1 set/**Twisting crunch** (done until failure)
- 1 set/**Twisting leg thrust** (done until failure)
- 1 set/**V-up with a twist** (done until failure)

Days 2 + 4 (Rest 45 seconds between sets)

- 4 sets/**Squat** (8–12 reps)
- 4 sets/**Deadlift** (8–12 reps)
- 4 sets/**Lunge** (8–12 reps)
- 3 sets/**Bent-over row** (8–12 reps)
- 3 sets/**Lat pulldown** (8–12 reps)
- 3 sets/**Biceps curl** (8–12 reps)
- 3 sets/**Reverse curl** (8–12 reps)
- 3 sets/**Standing calf raise** (8–12 reps)
- 1 set/**Crunch** (done until failure)
- 1 set/**Reverse crunch** (done until failure)
- 1 set/**Side raise** (done until failure)

45/4

Your Instant COMPLETE-BODY Plan!

Day 1 (Rest 45 seconds between sets)

4 sets/Bench press
(12–15 reps; 8–12 reps; 6–8 reps; 6–8 reps)

3 sets/Incline fly
(12–15 reps; 8–12 reps; 6–8 reps)

3 sets/Decline press
(12–15 reps; 8–12 reps; 6–8 reps)

4 sets/Seated shoulder press
(12–15 reps; 8–12 reps; 6–8 reps; 6–8 reps)

3 sets/Lateral raise
(12–15 reps; 8–12 reps; 6–8 reps)

2 sets/Shrug
(12–15 reps; 8–12 reps)

3 sets/Seated triceps extension
(12–15 reps; 8–12 reps; 6–8 reps)

3 sets/Triceps pushdown
(12–15 reps; 8–12 reps; 6–8 reps)

2 sets/Crunch
(each set done until failure)

2 sets/Reverse crunch
(each set done until failure)

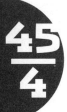

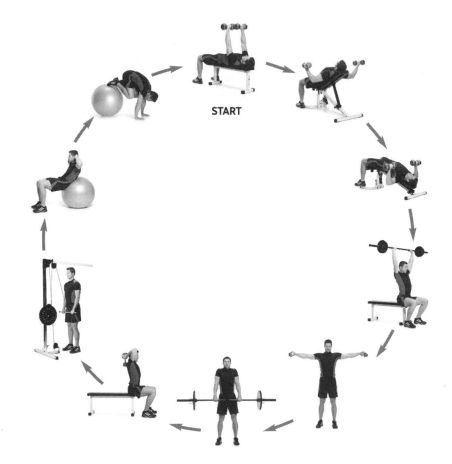

START

Day 2 (Rest 45 seconds between sets)

3 sets/**Squat**
(12–15 reps; 8–12 reps; 6–8 reps)

3 sets/**Lunge**
(12–15 reps; 8–12 reps; 6–8 reps)

2 sets/**Side lunge**
(12–15 reps; 8–12 reps)

4 sets/**Bent-over row**
(12–15 reps; 8–12 reps; 6–8 reps; 6–8 reps)

3 sets/**Lat pulldown**
(12–15 reps; 8–12 reps; 6–8 reps)

2 sets/**Upright row**
(8–12 reps; 6–8 reps)

3 sets/**Biceps curl**
(12–15 reps; 8–12 reps; 6–8 reps)

3 sets/**Reverse curl**
(12–15 reps; 8–12 reps; 6–8 reps)

2 sets/**Standing calf raise**
(12–15 reps; 8–12 reps)

2 sets/**Side raise**
(each set done until failure)

2 sets/**V-up with a twist**
(each set done until failure)

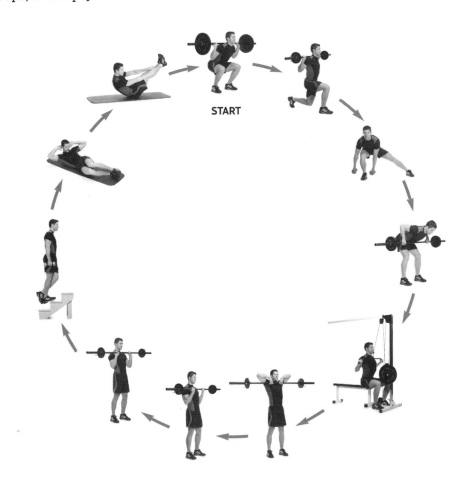

START

45/4

Your Instant **COMPLETE-BODY** Plan!—cont.

Day 3 (Rest 45 seconds between sets)

4 sets/**Bench press**
(12–15 reps; 8–12 reps; 6–8 reps; 6–8 reps)

3 sets/**Incline press**
(12–15 reps; 8–12 reps; 6–8 reps)

3 sets/**Chest fly**
(12–15 reps; 8–12 reps; 6–8 reps)

4 sets/**Seated shoulder press**
(12–15 reps; 8–12 reps; 6–8 reps; 6–8 reps)

3 sets/**Front raise**
(12–15 reps; 8–12 reps; 6–8 reps)

3 sets/**Bent-over reverse raise**
(12–15 reps; 8–12 reps; 6–8 reps)

3 sets/**Lying triceps press**
(12–15 reps; 8–12 reps; 6–8 reps)

2 sets/**One-arm triceps extension**
(12–15 reps; 8–12 reps)

2 sets/**Crunch**
(each set done until failure)

2 sets/**Reverse crunch**
(each set done until failure)

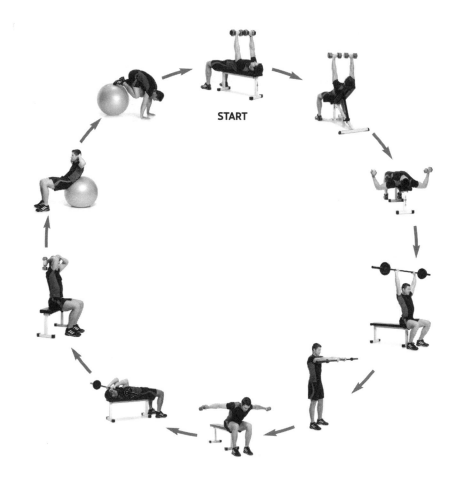

START

Day 4 (Rest 45 seconds between sets)

3 sets/**Front squat**
(12–15 reps; 8–12 reps; 6–8 reps)

3 sets/**Reverse lunge**
(12–15 reps; 8–12 reps; 6–8 reps)

4 sets/**One-arm row**
(12–15 reps; 8–12 reps; 6–8 reps; 6–8 reps)

3 sets/**Close-grip pulldown**
(12–15 reps; 8–12 reps; 6–8 reps)

3 sets/**Hammer curl**
(12–15 reps; 8–12 reps; 6–8 reps)

3 sets/**Preacher curl**
(12–15 reps; 8–12 reps; 6–8 reps)

1 set/**Wrist curl**
(8–12 reps)

1 set/**Wrist extension**
(8–12 reps)

3 sets/**Seated calf raise**
(12–15 reps; 8–12 reps; 8–12 reps)

2 sets/**V-up with a twist**
(each set done until failure)

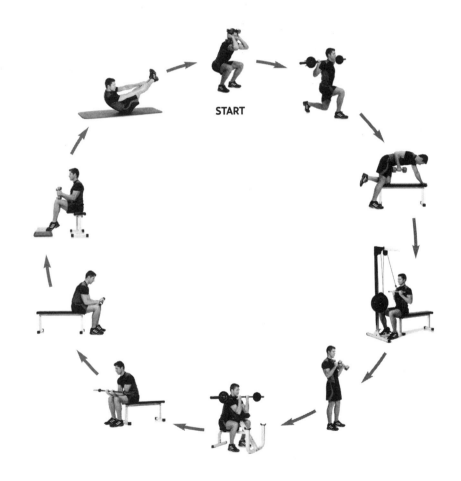

START

60 Minutes/4 Days a Week

Your Instant LEAN-BODY Plan!

60/4

Days 1 + 3 (Rest 15 seconds between sets)

2 minutes of low-intensity cardiovascular exercise

3 sets/**Bench press** (12–15 reps)

2 sets/**Incline press** (12–15 reps)

2 sets/**Incline fly** (12–15 reps)

3 sets/**Seated shoulder press** (12–15 reps)

2 sets/**Lateral raise** (12–15 reps)

3 sets/**Seated triceps extension** (12–15 reps)

2 sets/**Kickback** (12–15 reps)

2 sets/**Twisting leg thrust** (each set done until failure)

2 sets/**Twisting toe touch** (each set done until failure)

30 minutes of medium-intensity cardio

3 minutes of low-intensity cardio

Days 2 + 4 (Rest 15 seconds between sets)

2 minutes of low-intensity cardiovascular exercise

4 sets/**Squat** (12–15 reps)

3 sets/**Lunge** (12–15 reps)

3 sets/**Bent-over row** (12–15 reps)

3 sets/**Lat pulldown** (12–15 reps)

2 sets/**Biceps curl** (12–15 reps)

2 sets/**Preacher curl** (12–15 reps)

2 sets/**Crunch** (each set done until failure)

2 sets/**Reverse crunch** (each set done until failure)

30 minutes of medium-intensity cardio

3 minutes of low-intensity cardio

Your Instant POWER Plan!

Days 1 + 3 (Rest 2 minutes between sets)

- ⚡ 4 sets/**Bench press** (6–8 reps)
- ⚡ 3 sets/**Incline press** (6–8 reps)
- ⚡ 4 sets/**Push press** (6–8 reps)
- ⚡ 3 sets/**Seated shoulder press** (6–8 reps)
- ⚡ 4 sets/**Dip** (6–8 reps)
- ⚡ 3 sets/**Triceps pushdown** (6–8 reps)
- ⚡ 1 set/**Crunch** (done until failure)
- ⚡ 1 set/**Reverse crunch** (done until failure)
- ⚡ 1 set/**V-up with a twist** (done until failure)

Days 2 + 4 (Rest 2 minutes between sets)

- ⚡ 5 sets/**Squat** (6–8 reps)
- ⚡ 5 sets/**Deadlift** (6–8 reps)
- ⚡ 3 sets/**Lunge** (6–8 reps)
- ⚡ 4 sets/**Bent-over row** (6–8 reps)
- ⚡ 3 sets/**Lat pulldown** (6–8 reps)
- ⚡ 2 sets/**Biceps curl** (6–8 reps)
- ⚡ 1 set/**Twisting crunch** (done until failure)
- ⚡ 1 set/**Twisting toe touch** (done until failure)

Your Instant MUSCLE Plan!

Days 1 + 3 (Rest 90 seconds between sets)

- 3 sets/**Bench press** (8–12 reps)
- 3 sets/**Incline fly** (8–12 reps)
- 3 sets/**Decline press** (8–12 reps)
- 3 sets/**Seated shoulder press** (8–12 reps)
- 3 sets/**Lateral raise** (8–12 reps)
- 3 sets/**Bent-over reverse raise** (8–12 reps)
- 2 sets/**Seated triceps extension** (8–12 reps)
- 2 sets/**Triceps pushdown** (8–12 reps)
- 2 sets/**Lying triceps extension** (8–12 reps)
- 1 set/**Twisting crunch** (done until failure)
- 1 set/**Twisting leg thrust** (done until failure)
- 1 set/**V-up with a twist** (done until failure)

Days 2 + 4 (Rest 90 seconds between sets)

- 3 sets/**Squat** (8–12 reps)
- 3 sets/**Deadlift** (8–12 reps)
- 2 sets/**Lunge** (8–12 reps)
- 3 sets/**Bent-over row** (8–12 reps)
- 2 sets/**Lat pulldown** (8–12 reps)
- 3 sets/**Biceps curl** (8–12 reps)
- 2 sets/**Reverse curl** (8–12 reps)
- 3 sets/**Standing calf raise** (8–12 reps)
- 1 set/**Wrist curl** (8–12 reps)
- 1 set/**Wrist extension** (8–12 reps)
- 1 set/**Crunch** (done until failure)
- 1 set/**Reverse crunch** (done until failure)
- 1 set/**Side raise** (done until failure)

60/4

▶ Your Instant COMPLETE-BODY Plan!

Day 1 (Rest 45 seconds between sets)

3 sets/**Bench press**
(12–15 reps; 8–12 reps; 6–8 reps)

3 sets/**Incline fly**
(12–15 reps; 8–12 reps; 6–8 reps)

3 sets/**Decline press**
(12–15 reps; 8–12 reps; 6–8 reps)

3 sets/**Seated shoulder press**
(12–15 reps; 8–12 reps; 6–8 reps)

3 sets/**Lateral raise**
(12–15 reps; 8–12 reps; 6–8 reps)

2 sets/**Shrug**
(12–15 reps; 8–12 reps)

3 sets/**Seated triceps extension**
(12–15 reps; 8–12 reps; 6–8 reps)

3 sets/**Triceps pushdown**
(12–15 reps; 8–12 reps; 6–8 reps)

1 set/**Crunch**
(done until failure)

1 set/**Reverse crunch**
(done until failure)

2 minutes of low-intensity cardiovascular exercise

15 minutes of medium-intensity cardio

3 minutes of low-intensity cardio

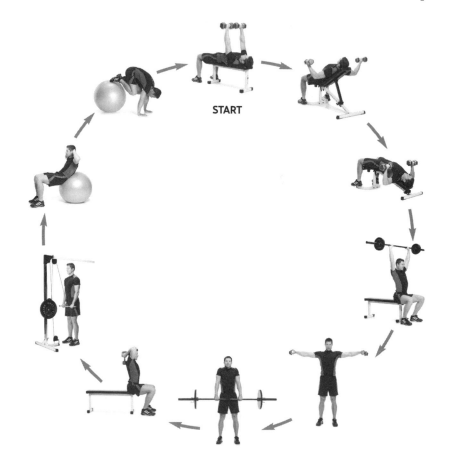

START

Day 2 (Rest 45 seconds between sets)

3 sets/**Squat**
(12–15 reps; 8–12 reps; 6–8 reps)

3 sets/**Lunge**
(12–15 reps; 8–12 reps; 6–8 reps)

2 sets/**Side lunge**
(12–15 reps; 8–12 reps)

3 sets/**Bent-over row**
(12–15 reps; 8–12 reps; 6–8 reps)

3 sets/**Lat pulldown**
(12–15 reps; 8–12 reps; 6–8 reps)

2 sets/**Upright row**
(8–12 reps; 6–8 reps)

3 sets/**Biceps curl**
(12–15 reps; 8–12 reps; 6–8 reps)

2 sets/**Reverse curl**
(8–12 reps; 6–8 reps)

2 sets/**Standing calf raise**
(12–15 reps; 8–12 reps)

1 set/**Side raise**
(done until failure)

1 set/**V-up with a twist**
(done until failure)

2 minutes of low-intensity cardiovascular exercise

15 minutes of medium-intensity cardio

3 minutes of low-intensity cardio

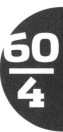

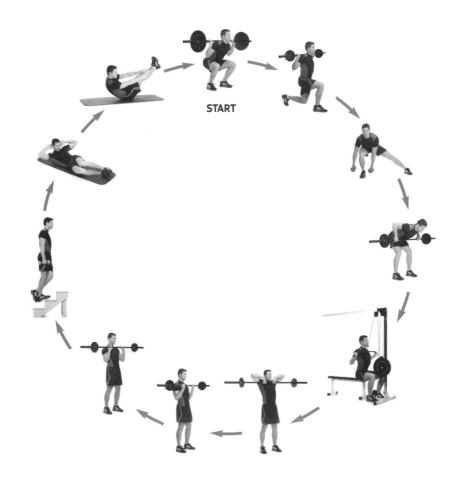

START

Your Instant COMPLETE-BODY Plan!—cont.

Day 3 (Rest 45 seconds between sets)

3 sets/**Bench press**
(12–15 reps; 8–12 reps; 6–8 reps)

3 sets/**Incline press**
(12–15 reps; 8–12 reps; 6–8 reps)

3 sets/**Chest fly**
(12–15 reps; 8–12 reps; 6–8 reps)

3 sets/**Seated shoulder press**
(12–15 reps; 8–12 reps; 6–8 reps)

3 sets/**Front raise**
(12–15 reps; 8–12 reps; 6–8 reps)

3 sets/**Bent-over reverse raise**
(12–15 reps; 8–12 reps; 6–8 reps)

3 sets/**Lying triceps press**
(12–15 reps; 8–12 reps; 6–8 reps)

3 sets/**One-arm triceps extension**
(12–15 reps; 8–12 reps)

3 sets/**Crunch**
(each set done until failure)

3 sets/**Reverse crunch**
(each set done until failure)

2 minutes of low-intensity cardiovascular exercise

15 minutes of medium-intensity cardio

3 minutes of low-intensity cardio

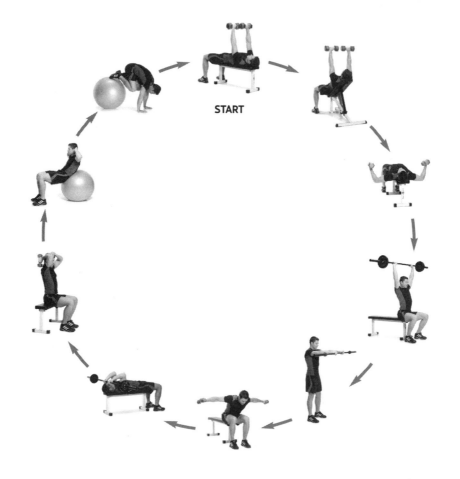

START

60/4

Day 4 (Rest 45 seconds between sets)

3 sets/**Front squat**
(12–15 reps; 8–12 reps; 6–8 reps)

3 sets/**Reverse lunge**
(12–15 reps; 8–12 reps; 6–8 reps)

3 sets/**One-arm row**
(12–15 reps; 8–12 reps; 6–8 reps)

3 sets/**Close-grip pulldown**
(12–15 reps; 8–12 reps; 6–8 reps)

3 sets/**Hammer curl**
(12–15 reps; 8–12 reps; 6–8 reps)

2 sets/**Preacher curl**
(8–12 reps; 6–8 reps)

1 set/**Wrist curl**
(8–12 reps)

1 set/**Wrist extension**
(8–12 reps)

2 sets/**Seated calf raise**
(12–15 reps; 8–12 reps)

2 sets/**V-up with a twist**
(each set done until failure)

2 minutes of low-intensity cardiovascular exercise

15 minutes of medium-intensity cardio

3 minutes of low-intensity cardio

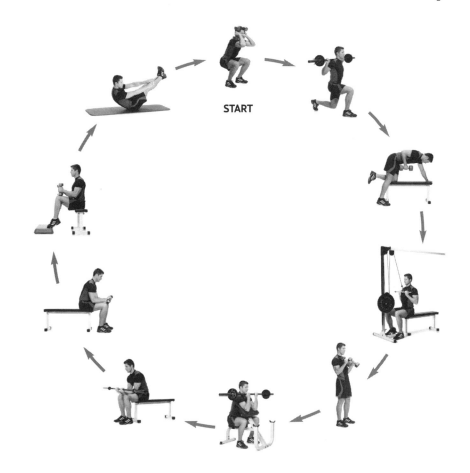

START

60
—
4

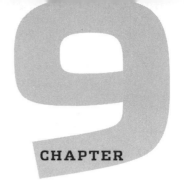

I Have 5 Days a Week

The 5-Day Edge

If you're reading this chapter, either you have high hopes of one day working out at this level, or you're already in good enough shape to handle this type of advanced schedule—especially if you're considering the 30-, 45-, or 60-minute routines in this chapter. Are you prepared to give your muscles the same 5-day-a-week attention you typically reserve for your day job? Are you serious about leaving your body no other choice but to step it up a notch and achieve results even faster than ever before? Have you been exercising for at least 6 months to a year?

Great! Then prepare yourself for the payoff!

Pushing yourself through a 5-day workout week means spending even more time breaking down your body, so it's left with no choice but to give you the physique you're looking for. If you're wondering what makes 5 days so effective, just flip back a chapter. The same benefits that come with the 4-day-a-week workouts apply to the routines in this section. But by adding just one more day, you'll end up training your muscles

the equivalent of an extra week per month. That means *you'll reach your muscular destination about 25 percent faster.*

Another day on your workout schedule also means another day of revving up your metabolism—the number of calories your body burns at any given moment to function throughout the day. Your body continues to burn calories at a higher rate for about 30 minutes to an hour after exercise, depending on how hard you pushed yourself. Revving your metabolism five times a week instead of four gives your body *an additional hour of calorie-burning time each week,* helping you lose more weight with the same routine.

Depending on your goals, that extra day of exercise can be the perfect time to add some cardiovascular training or stretching, without having to sacrifice a day of strength training. Some of the workouts in this chapter—mainly in the "complete-body plan" routines—utilize your fifth day of exercise to burn off excess calories, but that doesn't mean you can't use that fifth day for a cardio break in any of the other routines if you feel like trying it.

Here's How to Tweak Your Week

You'll notice that most of the routines in this chapter don't give you days by number—Day 1, Day 2, Day 3, for example—but by letters instead. Many of the routines are labeled "Workout A" and "Workout B." That's because you now have *two* ways you can use the routines on the following pages.

Your First Option

The first choice is to stick to the schedule and follow your workouts in order. You'll start the week with Workout A, but because you'll be exercising for an odd number of days, you'll end up finishing your week with Workout A as well. For example: Your 5-day schedule should look like this:

Day 1: Do Workout A

Day 2: Do Workout B

Day 3: Rest

Day 4: Do Workout A

Day 5: Do Workout B

Day 6: Do Workout A

Day 7: Rest

Because many of the workouts in this section are split routines, there's no need to worry about not giving your muscles enough rest from day to day. Still, if you do the math, you'll see that you're left training half of your body three times a week and the other half only twice each week. That's why it's crucial to start the second week the right way.

For the second week, you will need to start with Workout B and then end the week with Workout B.

Day 1: Do Workout B

Day 2: Do Workout A

Day 3: Rest

Day 4: Do Workout B

Day 5: Do Workout A

Day 6: Do Workout B

Day 7: Rest

You'll continue to alternate which workout you start with each week. If you're doing a 5-day plan for only 1 week, and you plan on changing your schedule the following week, then I recommend the second option (following) instead, to ensure that you'll train your muscles evenly.

Your Second Option

This second choice isn't nearly as complicated, and it gives you the freedom to decide how you spend your fifth day of exercise. Instead of ending the week with whichever workout you started with, you can use that day to rest, try one of the stretching programs in chapter 11, or turn back to chapter 5 for a 1-day-a-week program.

If you turn back to chapter 5, find a full-body plan that matches your goals—and that takes the same number of minutes as your other four workouts—and use that routine for your fifth day of exercise. Just remember that since all of the routines (except for some of the shorter "lean-body" plans that have you doing *only* cardio work) are full-body workouts, the muscles you trained during your last workout won't have had a solid 48 hours of recovery time. That's fine if you're planning to try this only once a month, but keep it in mind when you're doing exercises that train muscles you've hit the day before. To be on the safe side, try reducing the amount of weight you usually do in those exercises by 15 to 20 percent.

TIME TWEAKS!

Spend More Time . . . Eating Right around Your Workouts!

Putting in 5 days a week can take its toll on your body's energy levels as it is. That's why—whether you want to think about nutrition or not—it's important to know that *when* you eat can affect those levels as well. Here's how to plan your meals around the muscles you're trying to build.

Never eat fat 2 hours before a workout. Whenever you eat anything high in fat, your body pulls blood into your stomach to aid in the digestive process. That may be helpful for your stomach, but it's bad for your muscles, which need that oxygen-rich blood to train at their best. Fat takes the longest time to digest—about 3 to 4 hours—which leaves your muscles with less blood at their disposal for the entire

length of your workout and beyond. What to eat instead? Research has shown that eating a protein/carbohydrate meal several hours before working out causes a significant increase in growth hormone—the hormone your body uses to build muscle tissue.

Never eat *anything* right before a workout. If you're looking to really build muscle, save your appetite for later. Researchers at UCLA discovered that those who work out with partially digested food still in their stomachs suffer up to a 54 percent decrease in their body's natural production of growth hormone. In case you think that having an apple or some simple-sugar fruit beforehand won't be as big a deal, they also discovered that eating nothing but carbohydrates directly before a workout still causes a 24 percent drop in growth hormone production.

Always eat immediately after a workout. As I mentioned earlier in this book, exercise exhausts your body's supply of stored glycogen. That's why its first job after you exercise is replacing that glycogen so that your body has enough for your next workout. Your body processes glycogen twice as fast within the 15 to 45 minutes immediately following exercise. If you eat something as soon as you're finished working out, you can help replace glycogen even faster, so you have more energy for the next day's workout. If you don't, your body may look other places to find calories to convert, such as in the muscles you're trying to build.

You don't have to load up on a huge meal to keep your energy stores in check: Eating a piece of fruit or drinking a glass of milk 15 to 45 minutes after your workout will give your body enough carbohydrates to refuel, so it will leave your muscles alone.

10 Minutes/5 Days a Week

Your Instant LEAN-BODY Plan!

Days 1 + 3 + 5

1 minute of low-intensity cardiovascular exercise

8 minutes of high-intensity cardio

1 minute of low-intensity cardio

Days 2 + 4

1 minute of low-intensity cardiovascular exercise

**8 minutes of medium-/high-intensity cardio
(alternate between 30 seconds at a medium intensity
and 30 seconds at a high intensity)**

1 minute of low-intensity cardio

Your Instant POWER Plan!

Workout A (Rest 45 seconds between sets)

- 2 sets/**Power clean** (6–8 reps)
- 2 sets/**Bench press** (6–8 reps)
- 2 sets/**Push press** (6–8 reps)
- 2 sets/**Dip** (6–8 reps)

Workout B (Rest 45 seconds between sets)

- 3 sets/**Squat** (6–8 reps)
- 3 sets/**Deadlift** (6–8 reps)
- 2 sets/**Bent-over row** (6–8 reps)

Your Instant MUSCLE Plan!

Workout A (Rest 30 seconds between sets)

3 sets/**Bench press** (8–12 reps)
2 sets/**Seated shoulder press** (8–12 reps)
2 sets/**Seated triceps extension** (8–12 reps)
1 set/**Crunch** (done until failure—i.e., you can't do any more)

Workout B (Rest 30 seconds between sets)

3 sets/**Squat** (8–12 reps)
2 sets/**Bent-over row** (8–12 reps)
2 sets/**Biceps curl** (8–12 reps)
1 set/**Reverse crunch** (done until failure)

**10
5**

Your Instant **COMPLETE-BODY** Plan!

Day 1 (Rest 30 seconds between sets)

2 sets/**Bench press**
(8–12 reps)

2 sets/**Seated shoulder press**
(8–12 reps)

2 sets/**Seated triceps extension**
(8–12 reps)

2 sets/**Crunch**
(each set done until failure)

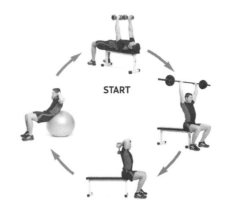

Day 2 (Rest 30 seconds between sets)

2 sets/**Squat**
(8–12 reps)

2 sets/**Lunge**
(8–12 reps)

2 sets/**Bent-over row**
(8–12 reps)

2 sets/**Biceps curl**
(8–12 reps)

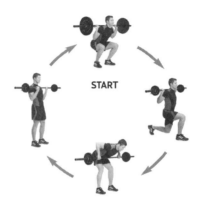

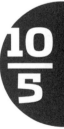

Your Instant COMPLETE-BODY Plan!—cont.

Day 3 (Rest 15 seconds between sets)

2 sets/**Incline press**
(12–15 reps)

2 sets/**Lateral raise**
(12–15 reps)

2 sets/**Triceps pushdown**
(12–15 reps)

2 sets/**Reverse crunch**
(each set done until failure)

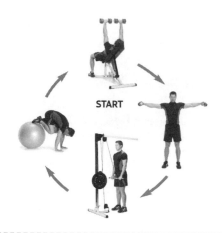

Day 4 (Rest 15 seconds between sets)

2 sets/**Front squat**
(12–15 reps)

2 sets/**Reverse lunge**
(12–15 reps)

2 sets/**Lat pulldown**
(12–15 reps)

2 sets/**Hammer curl**
(12–15 reps)

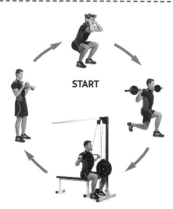

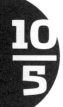

Day 5

1 minutes of low-intensity cardiovascular exercise

8 minutes of high-intensity cardio

1 minute of low-intensity cardio

20 Minutes/5 Days a Week

Your Instant LEAN-BODY Plan!

Days 1 + 3 + 5

2 minutes of low-intensity cardiovascular exercise

16 minutes of medium-intensity cardio

2 minutes of low-intensity cardio

Days 2 + 4

2 minutes of low-intensity cardiovascular exercise

16 minutes of medium-/high-intensity cardio (alternate between 60 seconds at a medium intensity and 60 seconds at a high intensity)

2 minutes of low-intensity cardio

Your Instant POWER Plan!

Workout A (Rest 60 seconds between sets)

- 4 sets/**Power clean** (6–8 reps)
- 3 sets/**Bench press** (6–8 reps)
- 3 sets/**Push press** (6–8 reps)
- 3 sets/**Dip** (6–8 reps)

Workout B (Rest 60 seconds between sets)

- 4 sets/**Squat** (6–8 reps)
- 4 sets/**Deadlift** (6–8 reps)
- 3 sets/**Bent-over row** (6–8 reps)
- 2 sets/**Biceps curl** (6–8 reps)

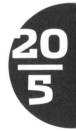

Your Instant MUSCLE Plan!

Workout A (Rest 30 seconds between sets)

3 sets/**Bench press** (8–12 reps)

2 sets/**Incline press** (8–12 reps)

3 sets/**Seated shoulder press** (8–12 reps)

2 sets/**Lateral raise** (8–12 reps)

3 sets/**Seated triceps extension** (8–12 reps)

2 sets/**Triceps pushdown** (8–12 reps)

1 set/**Crunch** (done until failure)

1 set/**Reverse crunch** (done until failure)

Workout B (Rest 30 seconds between sets)

3 sets/**Squat** (8–12 reps)

3 sets/**Lunge** (8–12 reps)

3 sets/**Bent-over row** (8–12 reps)

2 sets/**Lat pulldown** (8–12 reps)

2 sets/**Biceps curl** (8–12 reps)

2 sets/**Reverse curl** (8–12 reps)

1 set/**Crunch** (done until failure)

1 set/**Reverse crunch** (done until failure)

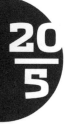

20 Minutes/5 Days a Week

Your Instant **COMPLETE-BODY** Plan!

Day 1 (Rest 30 seconds between sets)

3 sets/**Bench press**
(12–15 reps; 8–12 reps; 6–8 reps)

2 sets/**Incline press**
(8–12 reps; 6–8 reps)

3 sets/**Seated shoulder press**
(12–15 reps; 8–12 reps; 6–8 reps)

2 sets/**Lateral raise**
(8–12 reps; 6–8 reps)

3 sets/**Seated triceps extension**
(12–15 reps; 8–12 reps; 6–8 reps)

2 sets/**Triceps pushdown**
(8–12 reps; 6–8 reps)

1 set/**Crunch**
(done until failure)

1 set/**Reverse crunch**
(done until failure)

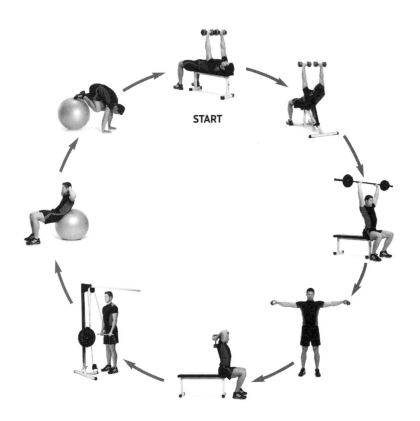

START

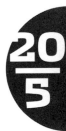

Your Instant **COMPLETE-BODY** Plan!—cont.

Day 2 (Rest 30 seconds between sets)

3 sets/**Squat**
(12–15 reps; 8–12 reps; 6–8 reps)

3 sets/**Lunge**
(12–15 reps; 8–12 reps; 6–8 reps)

3 sets/**Bent-over row**
(12–15 reps; 8–12 reps; 6–8 reps)

2 sets/**Lat pulldown**
(8–12 reps; 6–8 reps)

2 sets/**Biceps curl**
(8–12 reps; 6–8 reps)

2 sets/**Reverse curl**
(8–12 reps; 6–8 reps)

1 set/**Side raise**
(done until failure)

1 set/**V-up with a twist**
(done until failure)

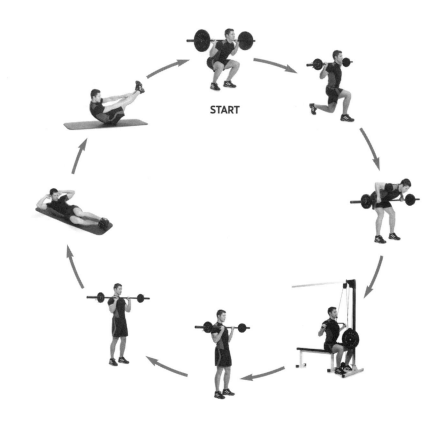

START

Day 3 (Rest 30 seconds between sets)

3 sets/**Bench press**
(12–15 reps; 8–12 reps; 6–8 reps)

2 sets/**Chest fly**
(8–12 reps; 6–8 reps)

3 sets/**Seated shoulder press**
(12–15 reps; 8–12 reps; 6–8 reps)

2 sets/**Bent-over reverse raise**
(8–12 reps; 6–8 reps)

3 sets/**Triceps pushdown**
(12–15 reps; 8–12 reps; 6–8 reps)

2 sets/**Dip**
(8–12 reps; 6–8 reps)

1 set/**Crunch**
(done until failure)

1 set/**Reverse crunch**
(done until failure)

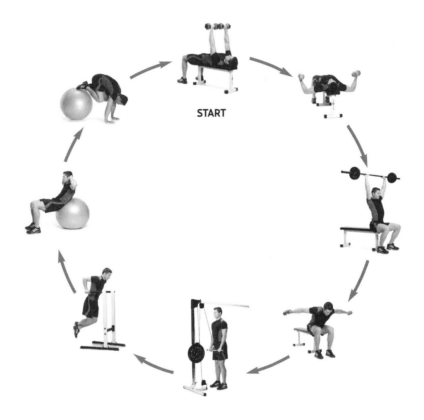

START

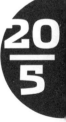

Your Instant **COMPLETE-BODY** Plan!—cont.

Day 4 (Rest 30 seconds between sets)

3 sets/**Front squat**
(12–15 reps; 8–12 reps; 6–8 reps)

3 sets/**Reverse lunge**
(12–15 reps; 8–12 reps; 6–8 reps)

2 sets/**One-arm row**
(8–12 reps; 6–8 reps)

2 sets/**Close-grip pulldown**
(8–12 reps; 6–8 reps)

2 sets/**Hammer curl**
(8–12 reps; 6–8 reps)

2 sets/**Preacher curl**
(8–12 reps; 6–8 reps)

1 set/**Side raise**
(done until failure)

1 set/**V-up with a twist**
(done until failure)

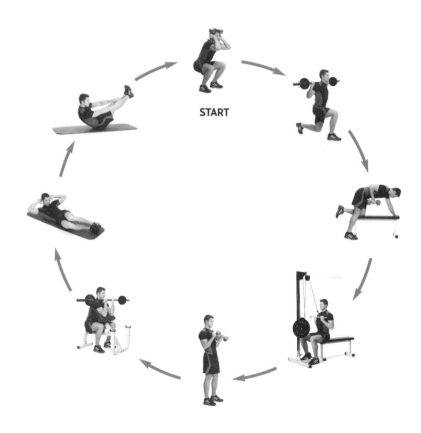

START

Day 5

2 minutes of low-intensity cardiovascular exercise

16 minutes of medium-intensity cardio

2 minutes of low-intensity cardio

30 Minutes/5 Days a Week

Your Instant LEAN-BODY Plan!

Days 1 + 3 (Rest 15 seconds between sets)

2 minutes of low-intensity cardiovascular exercise
2 sets/**Bench press** (12–15 reps)
2 sets/**Seated shoulder press** (12–15 reps)
2 sets/**Seated triceps extension** (12–15 reps)
2 sets/**Crunch** (each set done until failure)
16 minutes of medium-intensity cardio
2 minutes of low-intensity cardio

Days 2 + 4 (Rest 15 seconds between sets)

2 minutes of low-intensity cardiovascular exercise
2 sets/**Squat** (12–15 reps)
2 sets/**Lunge** (12–15 reps)
2 sets/**Bent-over row** (12–15 reps)
2 sets/**Biceps curl** (12–15 reps)
16 minutes of medium-intensity cardio
2 minutes of low-intensity cardio

Day 5

3 minutes of low-intensity cardiovascular exercise
25 minutes of medium-intensity cardio
2 minutes of low-intensity cardio

30/5

Your Instant POWER Plan!

Workout A (Rest 90 seconds between sets)

- 3 sets/**Bench press** (6–8 reps)
- 3 sets/**Incline press** (6–8 reps)
- 3 sets/**Decline press** (6–8 reps)
- 3 sets/**Seated shoulder press** (6–8 reps)
- 3 sets/**Dip** (6–8 reps)

Workout B (Rest 90 seconds between sets)

- 4 sets/**Squat** (6–8 reps)
- 4 sets/**Deadlift** (6–8 reps)
- 3 sets/**Lunge** (6–8 reps)
- 2 sets/**Bent-over row** (6–8 reps)
- 2 sets/**Biceps curl** (6–8 reps)

Your Instant MUSCLE Plan!

Workout A (Rest 30 seconds between sets)

4 sets/**Bench press** (8–12 reps)

3 sets/**Incline press** (8–12 reps)

2 sets/**Chest fly** (8–12 reps)

3 sets/**Seated shoulder press** (8–12 reps)

3 sets/**Lateral raise** (8–12 reps)

2 sets/**Bent-over reverse raise** (8–12 reps)

3 sets/**Seated triceps extension** (8–12 reps)

3 sets/**Triceps pushdown** (8–12 reps)

1 set/**Crunch** (done until failure)

1 set/**Reverse crunch** (done until failure)

Workout B (Rest 30 seconds between sets)

4 sets/**Squat** (8–12 reps)

3 sets/**Deadlift** (8–12 reps)

3 sets/**Lunge** (8–12 reps)

3 sets/**One-arm row** (8–12 reps)

3 sets/**Biceps curl** (8–12 reps)

3 sets/**Reverse curl** (8–12 reps)

3 sets/**Standing calf raise** (8–12 reps)

1 set/**Side raise** (done until failure)

1 set/**V-up with a twist** (done until failure)

$\dfrac{30}{5}$

30 Minutes/5 Days a Week

Your Instant **COMPLETE-BODY** Plan!

Day 1 (Rest 30 seconds between sets)

4 sets/**Bench press**
(12–15 reps; 8–12 reps; 6–8 reps; 6–8 reps)

3 sets/**Incline fly**
(12–15 reps; 8–12 reps; 6–8 reps)

3 sets/**Decline press**
(12–15 reps; 8–12 reps; 6–8 reps)

3 sets/**Seated shoulder press**
(12–15 reps; 8–12 reps; 6–8 reps)

3 sets/**Lateral raise**
(12–15 reps; 8–12 reps; 6–8 reps)

3 sets/**Seated triceps extension**
(12–15 reps; 8–12 reps; 6–8 reps)

3 sets/**Triceps pushdown**
(12–15 reps; 8–12 reps; 6–8 reps)

1 set/**Crunch**
(done until failure)

1 set/**Reverse crunch**
(done until failure)

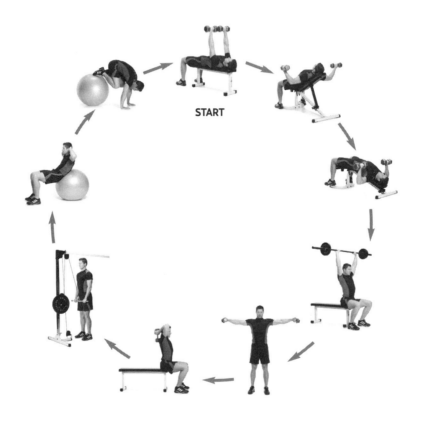

START

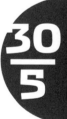

Your Instant **COMPLETE-BODY** Plan!—cont.

Day 2 (Rest 30 seconds between sets)

3 sets/**Squat**
(12–15 reps; 8–12 reps; 6–8 reps)

3 sets/**Lunge**
(12–15 reps; 8–12 reps; 6–8 reps)

2 sets/**Side lunge**
(12–15 reps; 8–12 reps)

3 sets/**Bent-over row**
(12–15 reps; 8–12 reps; 6–8 reps)

3 sets/**Lat pulldown**
(8–12 reps; 8–12 reps; 6–8 reps)

3 sets/**Biceps curl**
(8–12 reps; 8–12 reps; 6–8 reps)

3 sets/**Reverse curl**
(8–12 reps; 8–12 reps; 6–8 reps)

2 sets/**Standing calf raise**
(12–15 reps; 8–12 reps)

1 set/**Side raise**
(done until failure)

1 set/**V-up with a twist**
(done until failure)

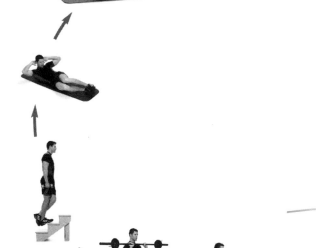

START

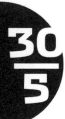

Day 3

2 minutes of low-intensity cardiovascular exercise

25 minutes of medium-intensity cardio

3 minutes of low-intensity cardio

Day 4 (Rest 30 seconds between sets)

4 sets/**Bench press**
(12–15 reps; 8–12 reps; 6–8 reps; 6–8 reps)

3 sets/**Chest fly**
(12–15 reps; 8–12 reps; 6–8 reps)

3 sets/**Seated shoulder press**
(12–15 reps; 8–12 reps; 6–8 reps)

3 sets/**Front raise**
(12–15 reps; 8–12 reps; 6–8 reps)

3 sets/**Bent-over reverse raise**
(12–15 reps; 8–12 reps; 6–8 reps)

3 sets/**Lying triceps press**
(12–15 reps; 8–12 reps; 6–8 reps)

2 sets/**One-arm triceps extension**
(12–15 reps; 8–12 reps)

1 set/**Crunch**
(done until failure)

1 set/**Reverse crunch**
(done until failure)

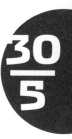

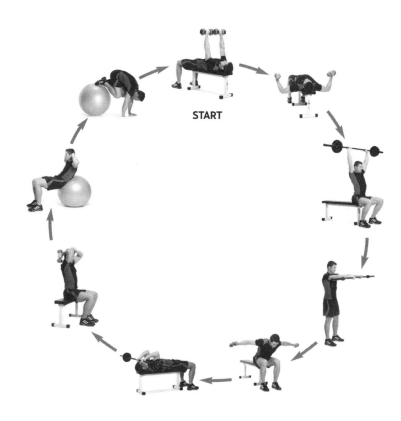

START

Your Instant **COMPLETE-BODY** Plan!—cont.

Day 5 (Rest 30 seconds between sets)

3 sets/**Front squat**
(12–15 reps; 8–12 reps; 6–8 reps)

3 sets/**Reverse lunge**
(12–15 reps; 8–12 reps; 6–8 reps)

3 sets/**One-arm row**
(12–15 reps; 8–12 reps; 6–8 reps)

3 sets/**Close-grip pulldown**
(8–12 reps; 8–12 reps; 6–8 reps)

3 sets/**Hammer curl**
(8–12 reps; 8–12 reps; 6–8 reps)

2 sets/**Preacher curl**
(8–12 reps; 6–8 reps)

1 set/**Wrist curl**
(8–12 reps)

1 set/**Wrist extension**
(8–12 reps)

2 sets/**Seated calf raise**
(12–15 reps; 8–12 reps)

1 set/**Side raise**
(done until failure)

1 set/**V-up with a twist**
(done until failure)

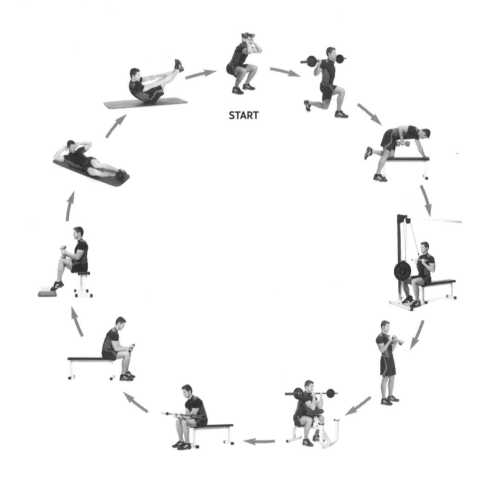

START

45 Minutes/5 Days a Week

Your Instant LEAN-BODY Plan!

Days 1 + 3 (Rest 15 seconds between sets)

2 minutes of low-intensity cardiovascular exercise

2 sets/**Bench press** (12–15 reps)

2 sets/**Chest fly** (12–15 reps)

2 sets/**Seated shoulder press** (12–15 reps)

2 sets/**Lateral raise** (12–15 reps)

2 sets/**Seated triceps extension** (12–15 reps)

2 sets/**Kickback** (12–15 reps)

2 sets/**Crunch** (each set done until failure)

2 sets/**Reverse crunch** (each set done until failure)

20 minutes of medium-intensity cardio

3 minutes of low-intensity cardio

Days 2 + 4 (Rest 15 seconds between sets)

2 minutes of low-intensity cardiovascular exercise

3 sets/**Squat** (12–15 reps)

3 sets/**Lunge** (12–15 reps)

2 sets/**Bent-over row** (12–15 reps)

2 sets/**Lat pulldown** (12–15 reps)

2 sets/**Biceps curl** (12–15 reps)

2 sets/**Crunch** (each set done until failure)

2 sets/**Reverse crunch** (each set done until failure)

20 minutes of medium-intensity cardio

3 minutes of low-intensity cardio

Day 5

5 minutes of low-intensity cardiovascular exercise

35 minutes of medium-intensity cardio

5 minutes of low-intensity cardio

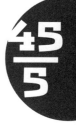

Your Instant POWER Plan!

Workout A (Rest 90 seconds between sets)

- 4 sets/**Bench press** (6–8 reps)
- 3 sets/**Incline press** (6–8 reps)
- 3 sets/**Decline press** (6–8 reps)
- 4 sets/**Seated shoulder press** (6–8 reps)
- 4 sets/**Dip** (6–8 reps)
- 3 sets/**Triceps pushdown** (6–8 reps)
- 1 set/**Crunch** (done until failure)
- 1 set/**Reverse crunch** (done until failure)

Workout B (Rest 90 seconds between sets)

- 5 sets/**Squat** (6–8 reps)
- 5 sets/**Deadlift** (6–8 reps)
- 3 sets/**Lunge** (6–8 reps)
- 3 sets/**Bent-over row** (6–8 reps)
- 3 sets/**Lat pulldown** (6–8 reps)
- 2 sets/**Biceps curl** (6–8 reps)
- 1 set/**Crunch** (done until failure)
- 1 set/**Reverse crunch** (done until failure)

Your Instant MUSCLE Plan!

Workout A (Rest 45 seconds between sets)

4 sets/**Bench press** (8–12 reps)
4 sets/**Incline press** (8–12 reps)
3 sets/**Decline press** (8–12 reps)
4 sets/**Seated shoulder press** (8–12 reps)
3 sets/**Lateral raise** (8–12 reps)
3 sets/**Bent-over reverse raise** (8–12 reps)
3 sets/**Seated triceps extension** (8–12 reps)
3 sets/**Triceps pushdown** (8–12 reps)
1 set/**Twisting crunch** (done until failure)
1 set/**Twisting leg thrust** (done until failure)
1 set/**V-up with a twist** (done until failure)

Workout B (Rest 45 seconds between sets)

4 sets/**Squat** (8–12 reps)
4 sets/**Deadlift** (8–12 reps)
4 sets/**Lunge** (8–12 reps)
3 sets/**Bent-over row** (8–12 reps)
3 sets/**Lat pulldown** (8–12 reps)
3 sets/**Biceps curl** (8–12 reps)
3 sets/**Reverse curl** (8–12 reps)
3 sets/**Standing calf raise** (8–12 reps)
1 set/**Crunch** (done until failure)
1 set/**Reverse crunch** (done until failure)
1 set/**Side raise** (done until failure)

45/5

45 Minutes/5 Days a Week

Your Instant COMPLETE-BODY Plan!

Day 1 (Rest 45 seconds between sets)

4 sets/Bench press
(12–15 reps; 8–12 reps; 6–8 reps; 6–8 reps)

3 sets/Incline fly
(12–15 reps; 8–12 reps; 6–8 reps)

3 sets/Decline press
(12–15 reps; 8–12 reps; 6–8 reps)

4 sets/Seated shoulder press
(12–15 reps; 8–12 reps; 6–8 reps; 6–8 reps)

3 sets/Lateral raise
(12–15 reps; 8–12 reps; 6–8 reps)

2 sets/Shrug
(12–15 reps; 8–12 reps)

3 sets/Seated triceps extension
(12–15 reps; 8–12 reps; 6–8 reps)

3 sets/Triceps pushdown
(12–15 reps; 8–12 reps; 6–8 reps)

2 sets/Crunch
(each set done until failure)

2 sets/Reverse crunch
(each set done until failure)

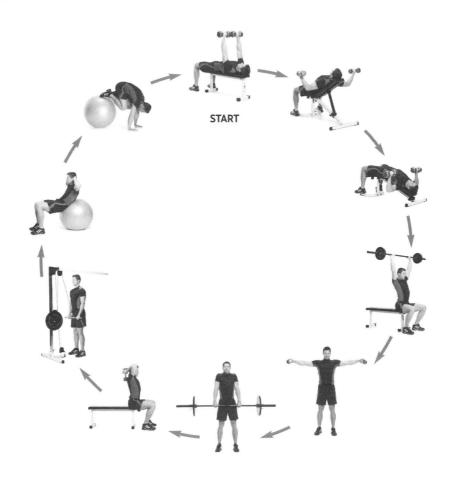

START

Your Instant **COMPLETE-BODY** Plan!—cont.

Day 2 (Rest 45 seconds between sets)

3 sets/**Squat**
(12–15 reps; 8–12 reps; 6–8 reps)

3 sets/**Lunge**
(12–15 reps; 8–12 reps; 6–8 reps)

2 sets/**Side lunge**
(12–15 reps; 8–12 reps)

4 sets/**Bent-over row**
(12–15 reps; 8–12 reps; 6–8 reps; 6–8 reps)

3 sets/**Lat pulldown**
(12–15 reps; 8–12 reps; 6–8 reps)

2 sets/**Upright row**
(8–12 reps; 6–8 reps)

3 sets/**Biceps curl**
(12–15 reps; 8–12 reps; 6–8 reps)

3 sets/**Reverse curl**
(12–15 reps; 8–12 reps; 6–8 reps)

2 sets/**Standing calf raise**
(12–15 reps; 8–12 reps)

2 sets/**Side raise**
(each set done until failure)

2 sets/**V-up with a twist**
(each set done until failure)

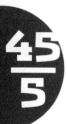

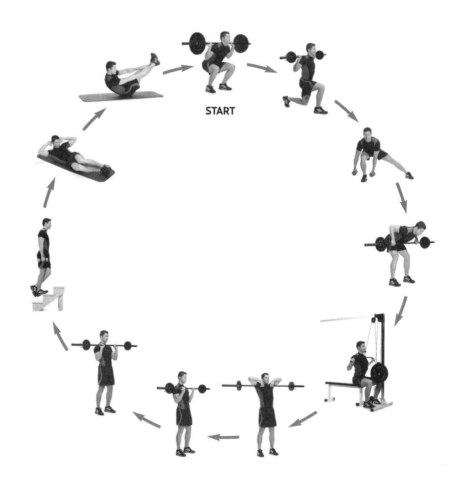

START

Day 3

5 minutes of low-intensity cardiovascular exercise

35 minutes of medium-intensity cardio

5 minutes of low-intensity cardio

Day 4 (Rest 45 seconds between sets)

4 sets/**Bench press**
(12–15 reps; 8–12 reps; 6–8 reps; 6–8 reps)

3 sets/**Incline press**
(12–15 reps; 8–12 reps; 6–8 reps)

3 sets/**Chest fly**
(12–15 reps; 8–12 reps; 6–8 reps)

4 sets/**Seated shoulder press**
(12–15 reps; 8–12 reps; 6–8 reps; 6–8 reps)

3 sets/**Front raise**
(12–15 reps; 8–12 reps; 6–8 reps)

3 sets/**Bent-over reverse raise**
(12–15 reps; 8–12 reps; 6–8 reps)

3 sets/**Lying triceps press**
(12–15 reps; 8–12 reps; 6–8 reps)

2 sets/**One-arm triceps extension**
(12–15 reps; 8–12 reps)

2 sets/**Crunch**
(each set done until failure)

2 sets/**Reverse crunch**
(each set done until failure)

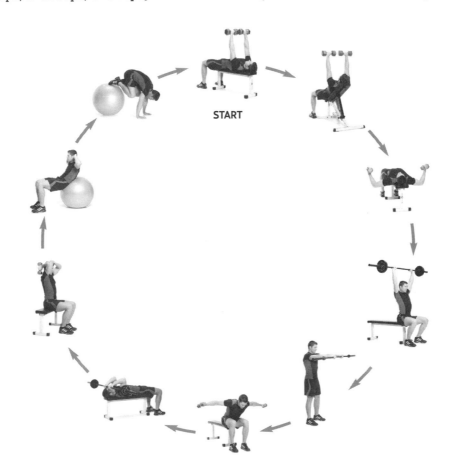

START

45/5

Your Instant **COMPLETE-BODY** Plan!—cont.

Day 5 (Rest 45 seconds between sets)

3 sets/**Front squat**
(12–15 reps; 8–12 reps; 6–8 reps)

3 sets/**Reverse lunge**
(12–15 reps; 8–12 reps; 6–8 reps)

4 sets/**One-arm row**
(12–15 reps; 8–12 reps; 6–8 reps; 6–8 reps)

3 sets/**Close-grip pulldown**
(12–15 reps; 8–12 reps; 6–8 reps)

3 sets/**Hammer curl**
(12–15 reps; 8–12 reps; 6–8 reps)

3 sets/**Preacher curl**
(12–15 reps; 8–12 reps; 6–8 reps)

1 set/**Wrist curl**
(8–12 reps)

1 set/**Wrist extension**
(8–12 reps)

3 sets/**Seated calf raise**
(12–15 reps; 8–12 reps; 8–12 reps)

2 sets/**V-up with a twist**
(each set done until failure)

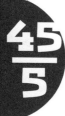

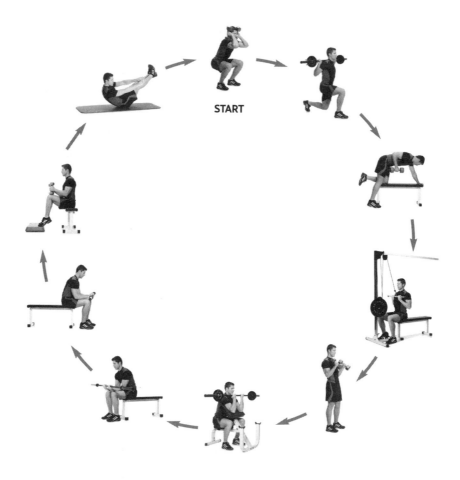

START

60 Minutes/5 Days a Week

Your Instant LEAN-BODY Plan!

Workout A (Rest 15 seconds between sets)

2 minutes of low-intensity cardiovascular exercise

3 sets/**Bench press** (12–15 reps)

2 sets/**Incline press** (12–15 reps)

2 sets/**Incline fly** (12–15 reps)

3 sets/**Seated shoulder press** (12–15 reps)

2 sets/**Lateral raise** (12–15 reps)

3 sets/**Seated triceps extension** (12–15 reps)

2 sets/**Kickback** (12–15 reps)

2 sets/**Twisting leg thrust** (each set done until failure)

2 sets/**Twisting toe touch** (each set done until failure)

30 minutes of medium-intensity cardio

3 minutes of low-intensity cardio

Workout B (Rest 15 seconds between sets)

2 minutes of low-intensity cardiovascular exercise

4 sets/**Squat** (12–15 reps)

3 sets/**Lunge** (12–15 reps)

3 sets/**Bent-over row** (12–15 reps)

3 sets/**Lat pulldown** (12–15 reps)

2 sets/**Biceps curl** (12–15 reps)

2 sets/**Preacher curl** (12–15 reps)

2 sets/**Crunch** (each set done until failure)

2 sets/**Reverse crunch** (each set done until failure)

30 minutes of medium-intensity cardio

3 minutes of low-intensity cardio

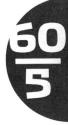

Your Instant POWER Plan!

Workout A (Rest 2 minutes between sets)

- 4 sets/**Bench press** (6–8 reps)
- 3 sets/**Incline press** (6–8 reps)
- 4 sets/**Push press** (6–8 reps)
- 3 sets/**Seated shoulder press** (6–8 reps)
- 4 sets/**Dip** (6–8 reps)
- 3 sets/**Triceps pushdown** (6–8 reps)
- 1 set/**Crunch** (done until failure)
- 1 set/**Reverse crunch** (done until failure)
- 1 set/**V-up with a twist** (done until failure)

Workout B (Rest 2 minutes between sets)

- 5 sets/**Squat** (6–8 reps)
- 5 sets/**Deadlift** (6–8 reps)
- 3 sets/**Lunge** (6–8 reps)
- 4 sets/**Bent-over row** (6–8 reps)
- 3 sets/**Lat pulldown** (6–8 reps)
- 2 sets/**Biceps curl** (6–8 reps)
- 1 set/**Twisting crunch** (done until failure)
- 1 set/**Twisting toe touch** (done until failure)

60 / 5

Your Instant MUSCLE Plan!

Workout A (Rest 90 seconds between sets)

3 sets/**Bench press** (8–12 reps)

3 sets/**Incline fly** (8–12 reps)

3 sets/**Decline press** (8–12 reps)

3 sets/**Seated shoulder press** (8–12 reps)

3 sets/**Lateral raise** (8–12 reps)

3 sets/**Bent-over reverse raise** (8–12 reps)

2 sets/**Seated triceps extension** (8–12 reps)

2 sets/**Triceps pushdown** (8–12 reps)

2 sets/**Lying triceps extension** (8–12 reps)

1 set/**Twisting crunch** (done until failure)

1 set/**Twisting leg thrust** (done until failure)

1 set/**V-up with a twist** (done until failure)

Workout B (Rest 90 seconds between sets)

3 sets/**Squat** (8–12 reps)

3 sets/**Deadlift** (8–12 reps)

2 sets/**Lunge** (8–12 reps)

3 sets/**Bent-over row** (8–12 reps)

2 sets/**Lat pulldown** (8–12 reps)

3 sets/**Biceps curl** (8–12 reps)

2 sets/**Reverse curl** (8–12 reps)

3 sets/**Standing calf raise** (8–12 reps)

1 set/**Wrist curl** (8–12 reps)

1 set/**Wrist extension** (8–12 reps)

1 set/**Crunch** (done until failure)

1 set/**Reverse crunch** (done until failure)

1 set/**Side raise** (done until failure)

60/5

Your Instant **COMPLETE-BODY** Plan!

Workout A (Rest 60 seconds between sets)

3 sets/**Bench press**
(12–15 reps; 8–12 reps; 6–8 reps)

3 sets/**Incline fly**
(12–15 reps; 8–12 reps; 6–8 reps)

2 sets/**Decline press**
(8–12 reps; 6–8 reps)

3 sets/**Seated shoulder press**
(12–15 reps; 8–12 reps; 6–8 reps)

3 sets/**Lateral raise**
(12–15 reps; 8–12 reps; 6–8 reps)

3 sets/**Seated triceps extension**
(12–15 reps; 8–12 reps; 6–8 reps)

2 sets/**Triceps pushdown**
(8–12 reps; 6–8 reps)

1 set/**Crunch**
(done until failure)

1 set/**Reverse crunch**
(done until failure)

2 minutes of low-intensity cardiovascular exercise

20 minutes of medium-intensity cardio

3 minutes of low-intensity cardio

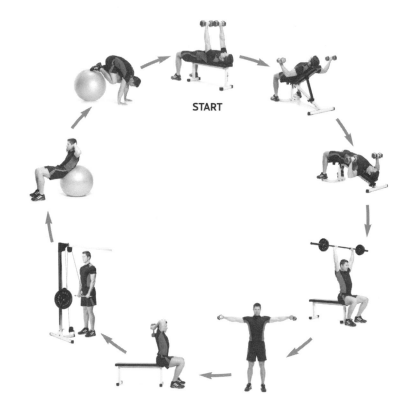

START

60/5

Workout B (Rest 60 seconds between sets)

3 sets/**Squat**
(12–15 reps; 8–12 reps; 6–8 reps)

3 sets/**Lunge**
(12–15 reps; 8–12 reps; 6–8 reps)

3 sets/**Bent-over row**
(12–15 reps; 8–12 reps; 6–8 reps)

3 sets/**Lat pulldown**
(12–15 reps; 8–12 reps; 6–8 reps)

3 sets/**Biceps curl**
(12–15 reps; 8–12 reps; 6–8 reps)

2 sets/**Reverse curl**
(8–12 reps; 6–8 reps)

2 sets/**Standing calf raise**
(12–15 reps; 8–12 reps)

1 set/**Side raise**
(done until failure)

1 set/**V-up with a twist**
(done until failure)

2 minutes of low-intensity cardiovascular exercise

20 minutes of medium-intensity cardio

3 minutes of low-intensity cardio

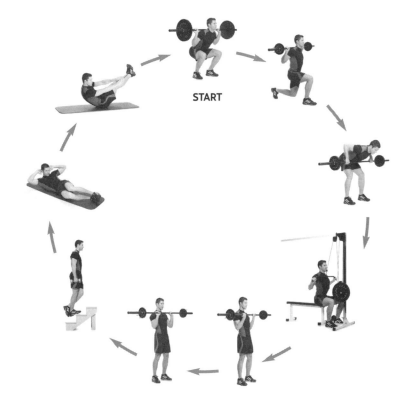

START

Your Instant **COMPLETE-BODY** Plan!—cont.

Workout C (Rest 60 seconds between sets)

3 sets/**Bench press**
(12–15 reps; 8–12 reps; 6–8 reps)

2 sets/**Incline press**
(8–12 reps; 6–8 reps)

2 sets/**Chest fly**
(12–15 reps; 8–12 reps)

3 sets/**Seated shoulder press**
(12–15 reps; 8–12 reps; 6–8 reps)

2 sets/**Front raise**
(12–15 reps; 8–12 reps)

2 sets/**Bent-over reverse raise**
(12–15 reps; 8–12 reps)

3 sets/**Lying triceps press**
(12–15 reps; 8–12 reps; 6–8 reps)

2 sets/**One-arm triceps extension**
(12–15 reps; 8–12 reps)

1 set/**Crunch**
(done until failure)

1 set/**Reverse crunch**
(done until failure)

2 minutes of low-intensity cardiovascular exercise

20 minutes of medium-intensity cardio

3 minutes of low-intensity cardio

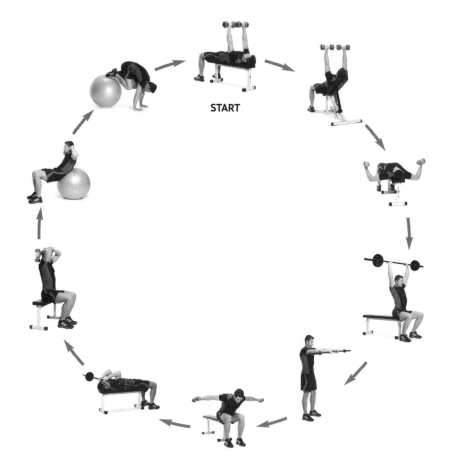

START

60
5

Workout D (Rest 60 seconds between sets)

3 sets/**Front squat**
(12–15 reps; 8–12 reps; 6–8 reps)

2 sets/**Reverse lunge**
(12–15 reps; 8–12 reps)

3 sets/**One-arm row**
(12–15 reps; 8–12 reps; 6–8 reps)

2 sets/**Close-grip pulldown**
(8–12 reps; 6–8 reps)

3 sets/**Hammer curl**
(12–15 reps; 8–12 reps; 6–8 reps)

2 sets/**Preacher curl**
(8–12 reps; 6–8 reps)

1 set/**Wrist curl**
(8–12 reps)

1 set/**Wrist extension**
(8–12 reps)

2 sets/**Seated calf raise**
(12–15 reps; 8–12 reps)

2 sets/**V-up with a twist**
(each set done until failure)

2 minutes of low-intensity cardiovascular exercise

20 minutes of medium-intensity cardio

3 minutes of low-intensity cardio

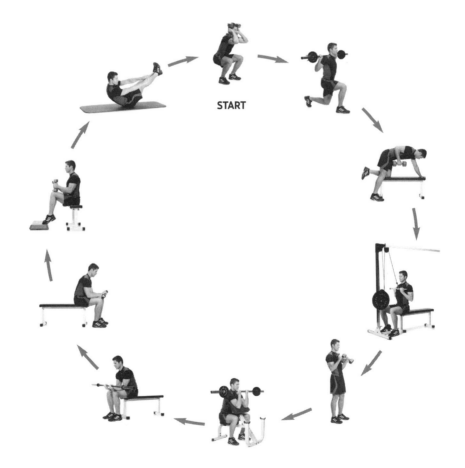

START

CHAPTER 10

I Have 6 Days a Week

The Six-Pack Advantage

With 6 days in your weekly arsenal, you now have more than enough time to focus your efforts on whichever muscles you really want to improve. Training your muscles to grow and reach new pinnacles of size, strength, and stamina requires isolating those areas with as many different exercises as possible. If you're serious about reshaping your muscles, you should do at least three or four exercises for larger muscle groups (the legs, chest, and back) and two or three exercises for smaller muscles (the arms, shoulders, abs, and calves). A 6-day schedule leaves you plenty of room to time-target those areas every single week.

Here's some more good news: If you exercise a minimum of 20 minutes per workout, you're on an intermediate level that's beyond what most people ever reach with their fitness goals. And if you exercise 6 days a week and 30 minutes a day or more, you can place yourself in the advanced category.

Here's How to Tweak Your Week

Six days' worth of workouts means you have far more choices to consider than usual.

There are many different schools of thought when it comes to how you should exercise during the week. Some advanced exercisers prefer to keep their full-body routines split in half and repeat both workouts three times a week. Other serious athletes opt to spread their entire workout across 6 days, focusing on just one or two muscle groups per session. But since the smartest way to work out is to use whatever keeps you injury-free (so you can exercise the next week, and the week after that!), the following routines are designed for maximum muscle recuperation between workouts.

Six days of training is a lot to ask of your muscles, even if you consider yourself an intermediate or advanced exerciser. That's why you'll be working each muscle group only twice a week: They'll get the break they need for growing.

Your First Option

Many of the routines on the next few pages will break up your muscles in the following order:

Day 1: Chest, shoulders, and triceps

Day 2: Back and biceps

Day 3: Legs

Day 4: Chest, shoulders, and triceps

Day 5: Back and biceps

Day 6: Legs

Day 7: Rest

The major differences between this program and the ones you may already have tried in chapters 8 and 9 is that, now, you'll be giving your legs their own separate workout. Dividing your muscles into three separate groups also means you'll have the same amount of time to exercise but fewer muscles to train during each workout. That means you can expect these routines to have an extra exercise or two per muscle group than you may be used to.

Your Second Option

You'll also notice that some of the workouts divide your muscles up differently from what you've seen up to now. Depending on your exercise goals, you may see routines that break down like so.

Day 1: Chest and back

Day 2: Shoulders and arms

TIME TWEAKS!

Spend More Time . . . Lowering Your Weights!

Lifting weights may forge a strong physique, but it's learning how to lower them that could decide between the body you currently have and the one you're hoping to create for yourself.

Quick lesson in anatomy!

When you lift a weight, a bar, or the like, you're contracting whichever muscles you're using to lift it. When your muscles contract, what they're *actually* doing is shortening themselves to get whatever body part they're attached onto—your arms, legs, torso, etc.—to move. When you lower a weight, you're lengthening the muscles, but they're still working hard for you. In fact, they're a lot stronger than you think at that moment.

Your muscles are actually about 20 percent stronger when you lengthen them than when you shorten them. For you, that means you can *technically* use more weight when doing an exercise—but only if all you do is lower it. What happens when you add more weight is that you overload your muscles more than usual, since more muscle fibers have to fire to handle the extra weight. The more fibers you can train within a workout, the faster you'll notice results and force your muscles to grow bigger and stronger.

Because of the demands that this *negative training* technique puts on your muscles, it's not meant for beginners. It also requires a little help—like a training partner. If you've got the experience and the assistance, then here are the rules.

Do all but the final set of an exercise, just as you normally would, saving this technique for the very last set of every exercise. For that final set, add about 10 to 20 percent more weight than you would typically handle, depending on the exercise. Have your partner assist you as much as possible during the lifting phase, then lower the weight on your own, at a slow, controlled pace. Try to slow the movement down so that it takes you at least 2 to 4 seconds to lower the weight. More time than that turns the exercise into an isometric movement that develops muscular endurance instead of size.

One final thought: Don't let the word *lift* make you believe that this technique applies only to movements that require you to lift a weight. It works not only with pushing exercises—such as bench presses, triceps pushdowns, shoulder presses, and squats—but also with curling or pulling exercises, such as rows, lat pulldowns, and biceps curls.

Day 3: Legs

Day 4: Chest and back

Day 5: Shoulders and arms

Day 6: Legs

Day 7: Rest

What most people never realize is that their muscles work in pairs. Whenever you contract a muscle—such as your biceps, for example—you have another muscle group directly behind it that's being stretched at the same time—in this case, your triceps. The same thing is true when you work any of your major and minor muscle groups. For instance . . .

Working your chest? You're indirectly stretching either your upper back and/or rear shoulders.

Working your upper back? You're indirectly stretching either your chest and/or front shoulders.

Working your lower back? You're indirectly stretching your abdominal muscles—and vice versa.

Working your biceps? You're indirectly stretching your triceps—and vice versa.

Working your quadriceps? You're indirectly stretching your hamstrings—and vice versa.

Now that you have the idea, here's why it's important to know. Pairing up opposing muscles with each other in the same workout—known as the "push-pull" method—can actually keep you injury-free, especially if you plan on putting in some exercise overtime.

You see, when you work opposing muscle groups together, you loosen both of them up indirectly as you exercise, which can prevent both sets of muscles from suffering from a strain or overstressing themselves. The "push-pull" routines in this section are designed to do just that, asking you to do one exercise for one muscle group, then another that works its opposite.

One example: You may do a bench press for your chest (where you'll push your arms away from your body), then a bent-over row (where you'll pull your arms in toward your chest). As

PAIRING UP OPPOSING MUSCLES WITH EACH OTHER IN THE SAME WORKOUT—KNOWN AS THE "PUSH-PULL" METHOD—CAN ACTUALLY KEEP YOU INJURY-FREE, ESPECIALLY IF YOU PLAN ON PUTTING IN SOME EXERCISE OVERTIME.

you strengthen your chest with the bench press, you're indirectly loosening up your back. So, by the time you move to the bent-over row, your upper back is already limber and more resistant to injury. As you perform the bent-over row, you're indirectly stretching your chest muscles—which may be tight from your last set of bench presses. As you alternate back and forth between exercises, the technique keeps your muscles from getting too tight as you exercise, leaving you with fewer pains and more gains.

Ready to give this a try? You should be. After all, if you have 6 days to offer, your muscles are counting on you to find new ways to challenge them that can keep them injury-free at the same time. These routines will make sure your muscles never quit—so your results never stop.

10 Minutes/6 Days a Week

Your Instant LEAN-BODY Plan!

All 6 Days

1 minute of low-intensity cardiovascular exercise

8 minutes of high-intensity cardio

1 minute of low-intensity cardio

Your Instant POWER Plan!

Days 1 + 4 (Rest 45 seconds between sets)

- ⚡ 2 sets/**Power clean** (6–8 reps)
- ⚡ 2 sets/**Bench press** (6–8 reps)
- ⚡ 2 sets/**Push press** (6–8 reps)
- ⚡ 2 sets/**Dip** (6–8 reps)

Days 2 + 5 (Rest 45 seconds between sets)

- ⚡ 3 sets/**Deadlift** (6–8 reps)
- ⚡ 3 sets/**Bent-over row** (6–8 reps)
- ⚡ 2 sets/**Biceps curl** (6–8 reps)

Days 3 + 6 (Rest 45 seconds between sets)

- ⚡ 3 sets/**Squat** (6–8 reps)
- ⚡ 3 sets/**Front squat** (6–8 reps)
- ⚡ 2 sets/**Lunge** (6–8 reps)

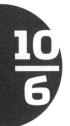

10
—
6

Your Instant MUSCLE Plan!

Days 1 + 4 (Rest 30 seconds between sets)

3 sets/**Bench press** (8–12 reps)

2 sets/**Seated shoulder press** (8–12 reps)

2 sets/**Seated triceps extension** (8–12 reps)

1 set/**Crunch** (done until failure—i.e., you can't do any more)

Days 2 + 5 (Rest 30 seconds between sets)

3 sets/**Lat pulldown** (8–12 reps)

2 sets/**Bent-over row** (8–12 reps)

2 sets/**Biceps curl** (8–12 reps)

1 set/**Reverse crunch** (done until failure)

Days 3 + 6 (Rest 30 seconds between sets)

4 sets/**Squat** (8–12 reps)

3 sets/**Lunge** (8–12 reps)

1 set/**Side raise** (done until failure)

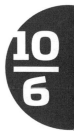

Your Instant COMPLETE-BODY Plan!

Days 1 + 4 (Rest 30 seconds between sets)

2 sets/**Bench press**
(8–12 reps; 6–8 reps)

2 sets/**Incline press**
(8–12 reps; 6–8 reps)

2 sets/**Seated shoulder press**
(8–12 reps; 6–8 reps)

2 sets/**Seated triceps extension**
(8–12 reps; 6–8 reps)

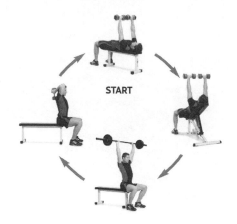

Days 2 + 5 (Rest 30 seconds between sets)

2 sets/**Bent-over row**
(8–12 reps; 6–8 reps)

2 sets/**Lat pulldown**
(8–12 reps; 6–8 reps)

2 sets/**Biceps curl**
(8–12 reps; 6–8 reps)

2 sets/**Crunch**
(each set done until failure)

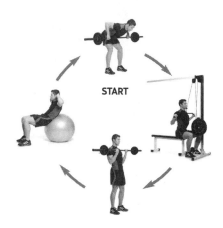

Days 3 + 6 (Rest 30 seconds between sets)

2 sets/**Squat**
(8–12 reps; 6–8 reps)

2 sets/**Lunge**
(8–12 reps; 6–8 reps)

2 sets/**Side lunge**
(8–12 reps; 6–8 reps)

2 sets/**Reverse crunch**
(each set done until failure)

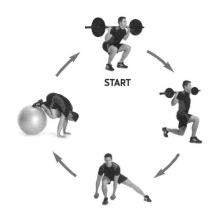

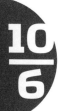

20 Minutes/6 Days a Week

Your Instant LEAN-BODY Plan!

Days 1 + 4

2 minutes of low-intensity cardiovascular exercise

16 minutes of high-intensity cardio

2 minutes of low-intensity cardio

Days 2 + 5

2 minutes of low-intensity cardiovascular exercise

16 minutes of medium-/high-intensity cardio (alternate between 60 seconds at a medium intensity and 60 seconds at a high intensity)

2 minutes of low-intensity cardio

Days 3 + 6

2 minutes of low-intensity cardiovascular exercise

16 minutes of high-intensity cardio

2 minutes of medium-intensity cardio

Your Instant POWER Plan!

Days 1 + 4 (Rest 60 seconds between sets)

- 3 sets/**Power clean** (6–8 reps)
- 4 sets/**Bench press** (6–8 reps)
- 3 sets/**Push press** (6–8 reps)
- 3 sets/**Dip** (6–8 reps)

Days 2 + 5 (Rest 60 seconds between sets)

- 4 sets/**Deadlift** (6–8 reps)
- 3 sets/**Bent-over row** (6–8 reps)
- 3 sets/**Lat pulldown** (6–8 reps)
- 3 sets/**Biceps curl** (6–8 reps)

Days 3 + 6 (Rest 60 seconds between sets)

- 4 sets/**Squat** (6–8 reps)
- 3 sets/**Front squat** (6–8 reps)
- 4 sets/**Lunge** (6–8 reps)
- 2 sets/**Standing calf raise** (6–8 reps)

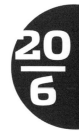

20/6

Your Instant MUSCLE Plan!

Days 1 + 4 (Rest 30 seconds between sets)

3 sets/**Bench press** (8–12 reps)

2 sets/**Incline press** (8–12 reps)

3 sets/**Seated shoulder press** (8–12 reps)

2 sets/**Lateral raise** (8–12 reps)

3 sets/**Seated triceps extension** (8–12 reps)

2 sets/**Triceps pushdown** (8–12 reps)

1 set/**Crunch** (done until failure)

1 set/**Reverse crunch** (done until failure)

Days 2 + 5 (Rest 30 seconds between sets)

4 sets/**Deadlift** (8–12 reps)

3 sets/**Bent-over row** (8–12 reps)

3 sets/**Lat pulldown** (8–12 reps)

3 sets/**Biceps curl** (8–12 reps)

2 sets/**Reverse curl** (8–12 reps)

1 set/**Crunch** (done until failure)

1 set/**Reverse crunch** (done until failure)

Days 3 + 6 (Rest 30 seconds between sets)

4 sets/**Squat** (8–12 reps)

3 sets/**Lunge** (8–12 reps)

3 sets/**Leg curl** (8–12 reps)

3 sets/**Leg extension** (8–12 reps)

1 set/**Crunch** (done until failure)

1 set/**Reverse crunch** (done until failure)

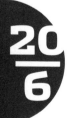

20/6

20 Minutes/6 Days a Week

Your Instant **COMPLETE-BODY** Plan!

Day 1 (Rest 30 seconds between sets)

3 sets/**Bench press**
(12–15 reps; 8–12 reps; 6–8 reps)

2 sets/**Incline press**
(8–12 reps; 6–8 reps)

3 sets/**Seated shoulder press**
(12–15 reps; 8–12 reps; 6–8 reps)

2 sets/**Lateral raise**
(8–12 reps; 6–8 reps)

3 sets/**Seated triceps extension**
(12–15 reps; 8–12 reps; 6–8 reps)

2 sets/**Triceps pushdown**
(8–12 reps; 6–8 reps)

1 set/**Crunch**
(done until failure)

1 set/**Reverse crunch**
(done until failure)

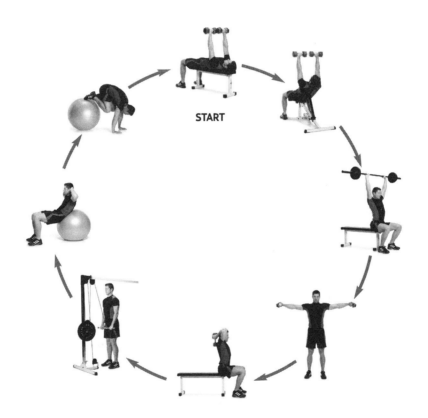

START

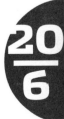

Your Instant **COMPLETE-BODY** Plan!—cont.

Day 2 (Rest 30 seconds between sets)

3 sets/**Squat**
(12–15 reps; 8–12 reps; 6–8 reps)

3 sets/**Lunge**
(12–15 reps; 8–12 reps; 6–8 reps)

3 sets/**Bent-over row**
(12–15 reps; 8–12 reps; 6–8 reps)

2 sets/**Lat pulldown**
(8–12 reps; 6–8 reps)

2 sets/**Biceps curl**
(8–12 reps; 6–8 reps)

2 sets/**Reverse curl**
(8–12 reps; 6–8 reps)

1 set/**Side raise**
(done until failure)

1 set/**V-up with a twist**
(done until failure)

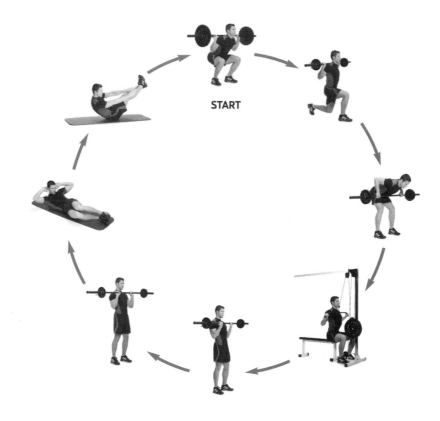

START

Day 3

2 minutes of low-intensity cardiovascular exercise

16 minutes of medium-intensity cardio

2 minutes of low-intensity cardio

Day 4 (Rest 30 seconds between sets)

3 sets/**Bench press**
(12–15 reps; 8–12 reps; 6–8 reps)

2 sets/**Chest fly**
(8–12 reps; 6–8 reps)

3 sets/**Seated shoulder press**
(12–15 reps; 8–12 reps; 6–8 reps)

2 sets/**Bent-over reverse raise**
(8–12 reps; 6–8 reps)

3 sets/**Triceps pushdown**
(12–15 reps; 8–12 reps; 6–8 reps)

2 sets/**Dip**
(8–12 reps; 6–8 reps)

1 set/**Crunch**
(done until failure)

1 set/**Reverse crunch**
(done until failure)

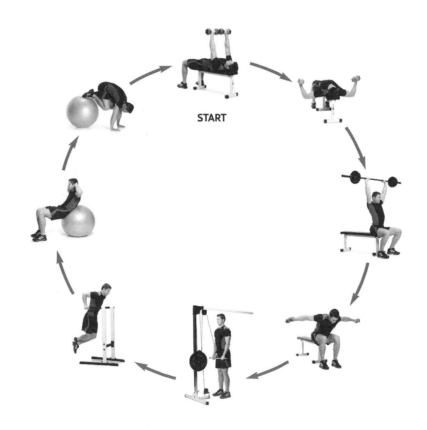

START

Your Instant COMPLETE-BODY Plan!—cont.

Day 5 (Rest 30 seconds between sets)

3 sets/**Front squat**
(12–15 reps; 8–12 reps; 6–8 reps)

3 sets/**Reverse lunge**
(12–15 reps; 8–12 reps; 6–8 reps)

2 sets/**One-arm row**
(8–12 reps; 6–8 reps)

2 sets/**Close-grip pulldown**
(8–12 reps; 6–8 reps)

2 sets/**Hammer curl**
(8–12 reps; 6–8 reps)

2 sets/**Preacher curl**
(8–12 reps; 6–8 reps)

1 set/**Side raise**
(done until failure)

1 set/**V-up with a twist**
(done until failure)

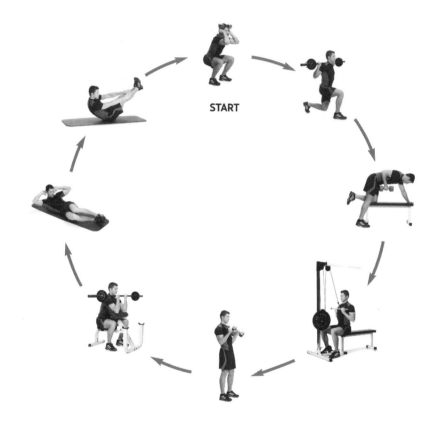

START

Day 6

2 minutes of low-intensity cardiovascular exercise

16 minutes of medium-intensity cardio

2 minutes of low-intensity cardio

30 Minutes/6 Days a Week

Your Instant LEAN-BODY Plan!

Days 1 + 4 (Rest 15 seconds between sets)

2 minutes of low-intensity cardiovascular exercise

2 sets/**Bench press** (12–15 reps)

2 sets/**Seated shoulder press** (12–15 reps)

2 sets/**Seated triceps extension** (12–15 reps)

2 sets/**Crunch** (each set done until failure)

16 minutes of medium-intensity cardio

2 minutes of low-intensity cardio

Days 2 + 5 (Rest 15 seconds between sets)

2 minutes of low-intensity cardiovascular exercise

2 sets/**Squat** (12–15 reps)

2 sets/**Lunge** (12–15 reps)

2 sets/**Bent-over row** (12–15 reps)

2 sets/**Biceps curl** (12–15 reps)

16 minutes of medium-intensity cardio

2 minutes of low-intensity cardio

Days 3 + 6

3 minutes of low-intensity cardiovascular exercise

25 minutes of medium-intensity cardio

2 minutes of low-intensity cardio

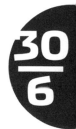

Your Instant POWER Plan!

Days 1 + 4 (Rest 90 seconds between sets)

- ⚡ 3 sets/**Bench press** (6–8 reps)
- ⚡ 3 sets/**Incline press** (6–8 reps)
- ⚡ 3 sets/**Decline press** (6–8 reps)
- ⚡ 3 sets/**Seated shoulder press** (6–8 reps)
- ⚡ 3 sets/**Dip** (6–8 reps)

Days 2 + 5 (Rest 90 seconds between sets)

- ⚡ 4 sets/**Deadlift** (6–8 reps)
- ⚡ 3 sets/**Bent-over row** (6–8 reps)
- ⚡ 3 sets/**Lat pulldown** (6–8 reps)
- ⚡ 3 sets/**Close-grip pulldown** (6–8 reps)
- ⚡ 2 sets/**Biceps curl** (6–8 reps)

Days 3 + 6 (Rest 90 seconds between sets)

- ⚡ 5 sets/**Squat** (6–8 reps)
- ⚡ 3 sets/**Lunge** (6–8 reps)
- ⚡ 3 sets/**Front squat** (6–8 reps)
- ⚡ 2 sets/**Leg curl** (6–8 reps)
- ⚡ 2 sets/**Standing calf raise** (8–12 reps)

30/6

Your Instant MUSCLE Plan!

Days 1 + 4 (Rest 45 seconds between sets)

3 sets/**Bench press** (8–12 reps)

3 sets/**Incline press** (8–12 reps)

2 sets/**Chest fly** (8–12 reps)

3 sets/**Seated shoulder press** (8–12 reps)

2 sets/**Lateral raise** (8–12 reps)

2 sets/**Bent-over reverse raise** (8–12 reps)

2 sets/**Seated triceps extension** (8–12 reps)

2 sets/**Triceps pushdown** (8–12 reps)

1 set/**Crunch** (done until failure)

1 set/**Twisting leg thrust** (done until failure)

Days 2 + 5 (Rest 45 seconds between sets)

3 sets/**Deadlift** (8–12 reps)

3 sets/**Bent-over row** (8–12 reps)

3 sets/**Lat pulldown** (8–12 reps)

3 sets/**Close-grip pulldown** (8–12 reps)

3 sets/**Biceps curl** (8–12 reps)

3 sets/**Reverse curl** (8–12 reps)

3 sets/**Side raise** (each set done until failure)

3 sets/**V-up with a twist** (each set done until failure)

Days 3 + 6 (Rest 45 seconds between sets)

5 sets/**Squat** (8–12 reps)

4 sets/**Reverse lunge** (8–12 reps)

3 sets/**Leg extension** (8–12 reps)

3 sets/**Leg curl** (8–12 reps)

3 sets/**Standing calf raise** (8–12 reps)

1 set/**Reverse crunch** (done until failure)

1 set/**Twisting crunch** (done until failure)

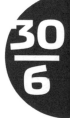

Your Instant COMPLETE-BODY Plan!

Day 1 (Rest 45 seconds between sets)

3 sets/**Bench press**
(12–15 reps; 8–12 reps; 6–8 reps)

3 sets/**Incline press**
(12–15 reps; 8–12 reps; 6–8 reps)

3 sets/**Seated shoulder press**
(12–15 reps; 8–12 reps; 6–8 reps)

3 sets/**Lateral raise**
(12–15 reps; 8–12 reps; 6–8 reps)

3 sets/**Seated triceps extension**
(12–15 reps; 8–12 reps; 6–8 reps)

3 sets/**Triceps pushdown**
(12–15 reps; 8–12 reps; 6–8 reps)

1 set/**Crunch**
(done until failure)

1 set/**Reverse crunch**
(done until failure)

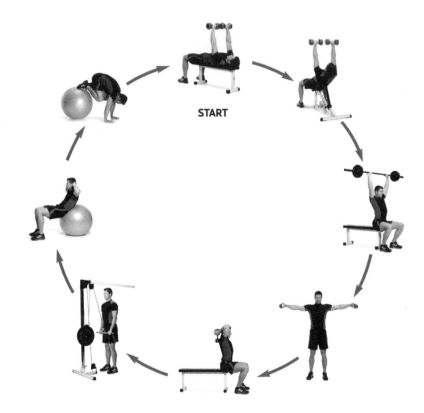

START

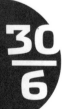

Day 2 (Rest 45 seconds between sets)

4 sets/Squat
(12–15 reps; 8–12 reps; 6–8 reps; 6–8 reps)

3 sets/Lunge
(12–15 reps; 8–12 reps; 6–8 reps)

3 sets/Bent-over row
(12–15 reps; 8–12 reps; 6–8 reps)

3 sets/Lat pulldown
(12–15 reps; 8–12 reps; 6–8 reps)

3 sets/Biceps curl
(12–15 reps; 8–12 reps; 6–8 reps)

2 sets/Reverse curl
(8–12 reps; 6–8 reps)

1 set/Side raise
(done until failure)

1 set/V-up with a twist
(done until failure)

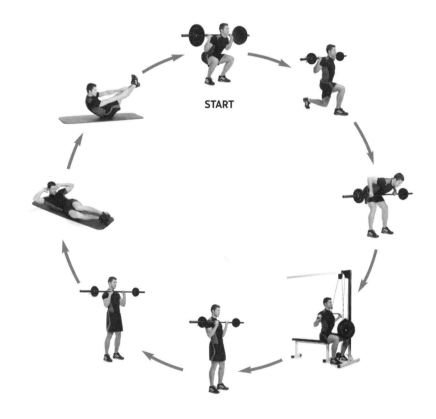

START

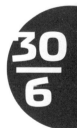

Your Instant **COMPLETE-BODY** Plan!—cont.

Day 3

2 minutes of low-intensity cardiovascular
exercise

25 minutes of high-intensity cardio

3 minutes of low-intensity cardio

Day 4 (Rest 45 seconds between sets)

3 sets/**Bench press**
(12–15 reps; 8–12 reps; 6–8 reps)

3 sets/**Chest fly**
(12–15 reps; 8–12 reps; 6–8 reps)

3 sets/**Seated shoulder press**
(12–15 reps; 8–12 reps; 6–8 reps)

3 sets/**Bent-over reverse raise**
(12–15 reps; 8–12 reps; 6–8 reps)

3 sets/**Triceps pushdown**
(12–15 reps; 8–12 reps; 6–8 reps)

3 sets/**Dip**
(12–15 reps; 8–12 reps; 6–8 reps)

1 set/**Crunch**
(done until failure)

1 set/**Reverse crunch**
(done until failure)

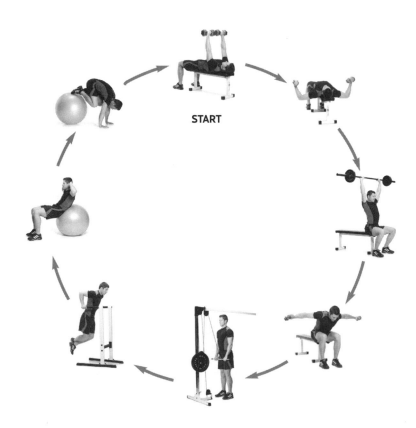

START

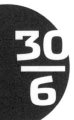

Day 5 (Rest 45 seconds between sets)

4 sets/**Front squat**
(12–15 reps; 8–12 reps; 6–8 reps; 6–8 reps)

3 sets/**Reverse lunge**
(12–15 reps; 8–12 reps; 6–8 reps)

2 sets/**One-arm row**
(8–12 reps; 6–8 reps)

2 sets/**Close-grip pulldown**
(8–12 reps; 6–8 reps)

3 sets/**Hammer curl**
(12–15 reps; 8–12 reps; 6–8 reps)

2 sets/**Preacher curl**
(8–12 reps; 6–8 reps)

1 set/**Side raise**
(done until failure)

1 set/**V-up with a twist**
(done until failure)

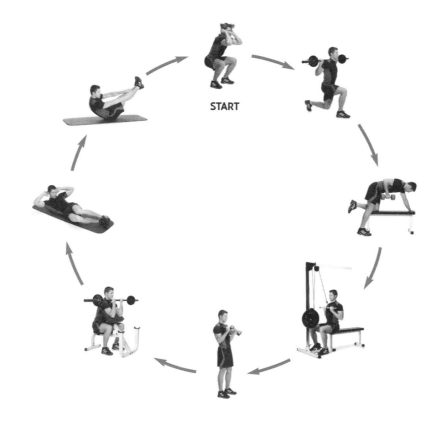

START

Day 6

2 minutes of low-intensity cardiovascular exercise

25 minutes of medium-intensity cardio

3 minutes of low-intensity cardio

30/6

45 Minutes/6 Days a Week

Your Instant LEAN-BODY Plan!

Days 1 + 4 (Rest 15 seconds between sets)

2 minutes of low-intensity cardiovascular exercise

2 sets/**Bench press** (12–15 reps)

2 sets/**Chest fly** (12–15 reps)

2 sets/**Seated shoulder press** (12–15 reps)

2 sets/**Seated triceps extension** (12–15 reps)

30 minutes of medium-intensity cardio

3 minutes of low-intensity cardio

Days 2 + 5 (Rest 15 seconds between sets)

2 minutes of low-intensity cardiovascular exercise

2 sets/**Bent-over row** (12–15 reps)

2 sets/**Lat pulldown** (12–15 reps)

2 sets/**Biceps curl** (12–15 reps)

1 set/**V-up with a twist** (done until failure)

30 minutes of medium-intensity cardio

3 minutes of low-intensity cardio

Days 3 + 6 (Rest 15 seconds between sets)

2 minutes of low-intensity cardiovascular exercise

3 sets/**Squat** (12–15 reps)

3 sets/**Lunge** (12–15 reps)

2 sets/**Twisting toe touch** (each set done until failure)

30 minutes of medium-intensity cardio

3 minutes of low-intensity cardio

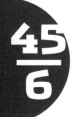

Your Instant POWER Plan!

Days 1 + 4 (Rest 90 seconds between sets)

- ⚡ 4 sets/**Bench press** (6–8 reps)
- ⚡ 3 sets/**Incline press** (6–8 reps)
- ⚡ 3 sets/**Decline press** (6–8 reps)
- ⚡ 4 sets/**Seated shoulder press** (6–8 reps)
- ⚡ 4 sets/**Dip** (6–8 reps)
- ⚡ 3 sets/**Triceps pushdown** (6–8 reps)
- ⚡ 1 set/**Crunch** (done until failure)
- ⚡ 1 set/**Reverse crunch** (done until failure)

Days 2 + 5 (Rest 90 seconds between sets)

- ⚡ 5 sets/**Deadlift** (6–8 reps)
- ⚡ 4 sets/**Bent-over row** (6–8 reps)
- ⚡ 3 sets/**Lat pulldown** (6–8 reps)
- ⚡ 3 sets/**Upright row** (6–8 reps)
- ⚡ 3 sets/**Biceps curl** (6–8 reps)
- ⚡ 3 sets/**Hammer curl** (6–8 reps)
- ⚡ 1 set/**Crunch** (done until failure)
- ⚡ 1 set/**Reverse crunch** (done until failure)

Days 3 + 6 (Rest 90 seconds between sets)

- ⚡ 5 sets/**Squat** (6–8 reps)
- ⚡ 4 sets/**Lunge** (6–8 reps)
- ⚡ 4 sets/**Leg extension** (6–8 reps)
- ⚡ 4 sets/**Leg curl** (6–8 reps)
- ⚡ 4 sets/**Standing calf raise** (8–12 reps)
- ⚡ 1 set/**Crunch** (done until failure)
- ⚡ 1 set/**Reverse crunch** (done until failure)

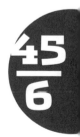

Your Instant MUSCLE Plan!

Days 1 + 4 (Rest 45 seconds between sets)

Push-pull superset: 4 sets/**Bent-over row** (8–12 reps)
+ 4 sets/**Bench press** (8–12 reps)

Push-pull superset: 4 sets/**Lat pulldown** (8–12 reps)
+ 4 sets/**Incline press** (8–12 reps)

Push-pull superset: 3 sets/**Upright row** (8–12 reps)
+ 3 sets/**Decline press** (8–12 reps)

3 sets/**Pullover** (8–12 reps)

2 sets/**Crunch** (each set done until failure)

2 sets/**Reverse crunch** (each set done until failure)

Days 2 + 5 (Rest 45 seconds between all sets)

4 sets/**Seated shoulder press** (8–12 reps)

3 sets/**Front raise** (8–12 reps)

3 sets/**Lateral raise** (8–12 reps)

3 sets/**Bent-over reverse raise** (8–12 reps)

Push-pull superset: 3 sets/**Biceps curl** (8–12 reps)
+ 3 sets/**Seated triceps extension** (8–12 reps)

Push-pull superset: 2 sets/**Hammer curl** (8–12 reps)
+ 2 sets/**Lying triceps press** (8–12 reps)

Push-pull superset: 2 sets/**Reverse curl** (8–12 reps)
+ 2 sets/**Triceps pushdown** (8–12 reps)

1 set/**Twisting crunch** (done until failure)

1 set/**Twisting leg thrust** (done until failure)

1 set/**V-up with a twist** (done until failure)

Days 3 + 6 (Rest 45 seconds between sets)

Push-pull superset: 4 sets/**Lunge** (8–12 reps)
+ 4 sets/**Squat** (8–12 reps)

Push-pull superset: 2 sets/**Reverse lunge** (8–12 reps)
+ 2 sets/**Front squat** (8–12 reps)

Push-pull superset: 2 sets/**Good morning** (8–12 reps)
+ 2 sets/**Side lunge** (8–12 reps)

Push-pull superset: 2 sets/**Leg curl** (8–12 reps)
+ 2 sets/**Leg extension** (8–12 reps)

Push-pull superset: 2 sets/**Standing calf raise** (8–12 reps)
+ 2 sets/**Seated calf raise** (8–12 reps)

1 set/**Crunch** (done until failure)

1 set/**Reverse crunch** (done until failure)

1 set/**Side raise** (done until failure)

*For supersets, do 1 set of the first exercise, then 1 set of the second. Alternate between both exercises until you've completed all your sets.

45/6

Your Instant COMPLETE-BODY Plan!

Day 1 (Rest 60 seconds between sets)

4 sets/**Bench press**
(12–15 reps; 8–12 reps; 6–8 reps; 6–8 reps)

3 sets/**Incline fly**
(12–15 reps; 8–12 reps; 6–8 reps)

3 sets/**Decline press**
(12–15 reps; 8–12 reps; 6–8 reps)

4 sets/**Seated shoulder press**
(12–15 reps; 8–12 reps; 6–8 reps; 6–8 reps)

3 sets/**Lateral raise**
(12–15 reps; 8–12 reps; 6–8 reps)

3 sets/**Seated triceps extension**
(12–15 reps; 8–12 reps; 6–8 reps)

3 sets/**Triceps pushdown**
(12–15 reps; 8–12 reps; 6–8 reps)

2 sets/**Crunch**
(each set done until failure)

2 sets/**Reverse crunch**
(each set done until failure)

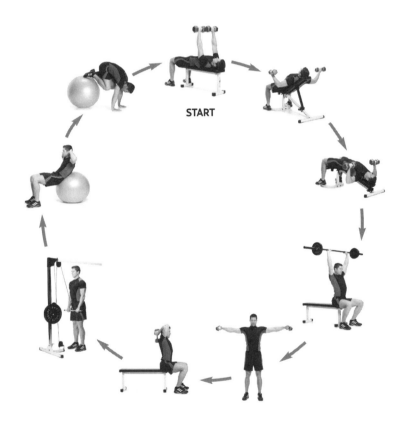

START

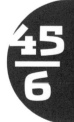

Your Instant **COMPLETE-BODY** Plan!—cont.

Day 2 (Rest 60 seconds between sets)

4 sets/**Squat**
(12–15 reps; 8–12 reps; 6–8 reps; 6–8 reps)

3 sets/**Lunge**
(12–15 reps; 8–12 reps; 6–8 reps)

4 sets/**Bent-over row**
(12–15 reps; 8–12 reps; 6–8 reps; 6–8 reps)

3 sets/**Lat pulldown**
(12–15 reps; 8–12 reps; 6–8 reps)

3 sets/**Pullover**
(12–15 reps; 8–12 reps; 6–8 reps)

3 sets/**Biceps curl**
(12–15 reps; 8–12 reps; 6–8 reps)

3 sets/**Reverse curl**
(12–15 reps; 8–12 reps; 6–8 reps)

2 sets/**Side raise**
(each set done until failure)

2 sets/**V-up with a twist**
(each set done until failure)

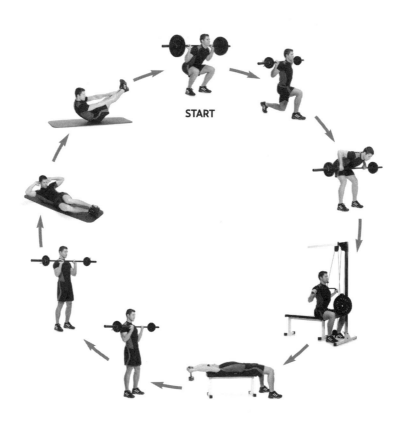

START

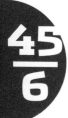

Day 3

5 minutes of low-intensity cardiovascular exercise

35 minutes of medium-intensity cardio

5 minutes of low-intensity cardio

Day 4 (Rest 60 seconds between sets)

4 sets/**Bench press**
(12–15 reps; 8–12 reps; 6–8 reps; 6–8 reps)

3 sets/**Incline press**
(12–15 reps; 8–12 reps; 6–8 reps)

3 sets/**Chest fly**
(12–15 reps; 8–12 reps; 6–8 reps)

4 sets/**Seated shoulder press**
(12–15 reps; 8–12 reps; 6–8 reps; 6–8 reps)

3 sets/**Bent-over reverse raise**
(12–15 reps; 8–12 reps; 6–8 reps)

3 sets/**Triceps pushdown**
(12–15 reps; 8–12 reps; 6–8 reps)

3 sets/**Dip**
(12–15 reps; 8–12 reps; 6–8 reps)

2 sets/**Crunch**
(each set done until failure)

2 sets/**Reverse crunch**
(each set done until failure)

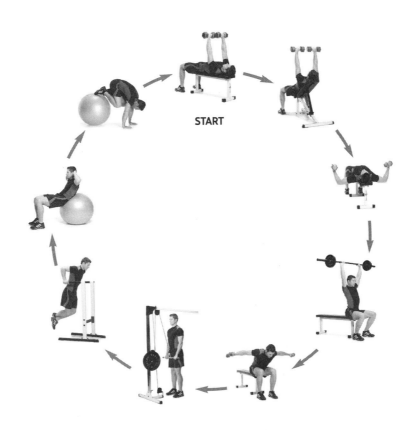

START

45/6

Your Instant **COMPLETE-BODY** Plan!—cont.

Day 5 (Rest 60 seconds between sets)

4 sets/**Front squat**
(12–15 reps; 8–12 reps; 6–8 reps; 6–8 reps)

3 sets/**Reverse lunge**
(12–15 reps; 8–12 reps; 6–8 reps)

3 sets/**One-arm row**
(12–15 reps; 8–12 reps; 6–8 reps)

3 sets/**Close-grip pulldown**
(12–15 reps; 8–12 reps; 6–8 reps)

3 sets/**Hammer curl**
(12–15 reps; 8–12 reps; 6–8 reps)

3 sets/**Preacher curl**
(12–15 reps; 8–12 reps; 6–8 reps)

1 set/**Wrist curl**
(8–12 reps)

1 set/**Wrist extension**
(8–12 reps)

2 sets/**Side raise**
(each set done until failure)

2 sets/**V-up with a twist**
(each set done until failure)

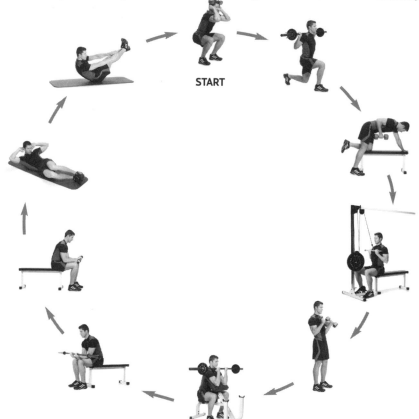

START

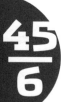

Day 6

5 minutes of low-intensity cardiovascular exercise

35 minutes of medium-/high-intensity cardio (alternate between 4 minutes at a medium intensity and 1 minute at a high intensity)

5 minutes of low-intensity cardio

60 Minutes/6 Days a Week

Your Instant LEAN-BODY Plan!

Days 1 + 4 (Rest 30 seconds between sets)

2 minutes of low-intensity cardiovascular exercise
3 sets/**Bench press** (12–15 reps)
2 sets/**Chest fly** (12–15 reps)
3 sets/**Seated shoulder press** (12–15 reps)
2 sets/**Lateral raise** (12–15 reps)
2 sets/**Seated triceps extension** (12–15 reps)
2 sets/**Kickback** (12–15 reps)
1 set/**V-up with a twist** (done until failure)
1 set/**Twisting toe touch** (done until failure)

30 minutes of medium-intensity cardio

3 minutes of low-intensity cardio

Days 2 + 5 (Rest 30 seconds between sets)

2 minutes of low-intensity cardiovascular exercise
4 sets/**One-arm row** (12–15 reps)
2 sets/**Lat pulldown** (12–15 reps)
3 sets/**Biceps curl** (12–15 reps)
2 sets/**Reverse curl** (12–15 reps)
1 set/**V-up with a twist** (done until failure)
1 set/**Twisting toe touch** (done until failure)

30 minutes of medium-intensity cardio

3 minutes of low-intensity cardio

Days 3 + 6 (Rest 30 seconds between sets)

2 minutes of low-intensity cardiovascular exercise
3 sets/**Squat** (12–15 reps)
3 sets/**Lunge** (12–15 reps)
3 sets/**Front squat** (12–15 reps)
3 sets/**Reverse lunge** (12–15 reps)
2 sets/**V-up with a twist** (each set done until failure)
2 sets/**Twisting toe touch** (each set done until failure)

30 minutes of medium-intensity cardio

3 minutes of low-intensity cardio

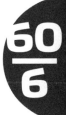

Your Instant POWER Plan!

Days 1 + 4 (Rest 2 minutes between sets)

- 4 sets/**Bench press** (6–8 reps)
- 3 sets/**Incline press** (6–8 reps)
- 3 sets/**Decline press** (6–8 reps)
- 5 sets/**Seated shoulder press** (6–8 reps)
- 4 sets/**Dip** (6–8 reps)
- 3 sets/**Triceps pushdown** (6–8 reps)
- 1 set/**Crunch** (done until failure)
- 1 set/**Reverse crunch** (done until failure)

Days 2 + 5 (Rest 2 minutes between sets)

- 5 sets/**Deadlift** (6–8 reps)
- 4 sets/**Bent-over row** (6–8 reps)
- 3 sets/**Lat pulldown** (6–8 reps)
- 3 sets/**Upright row** (6–8 reps)
- 4 sets/**Biceps curl** (6–8 reps)
- 3 sets/**Hammer curl** (6–8 reps)
- 1 set/**Crunch** (done until failure)
- 1 set/**Reverse crunch** (done until failure)

Days 3 + 6 (Rest 2 minutes between sets)

- 5 sets/**Squat** (6–8 reps)
- 4 sets/**Lunge** (6–8 reps)
- 4 sets/**Leg extension** (6–8 reps)
- 4 sets/**Leg curl** (6–8 reps)
- 4 sets/**Standing calf raise** (8–12 reps)
- 1 set/**Crunch** (done until failure)
- 1 set/**Reverse crunch** (done until failure)

60/6

Your Instant MUSCLE Plan!

Days 1 + 4 (Rest 90 seconds between sets)

*Push-pull superset:** 4 sets/**Bent-over row** (8–12 reps) + 4 sets/**Bench press** (8–12 reps)

*Push-pull superset:** 3 sets/**Lat pulldown** (8–12 reps) + 3 sets/**Incline press** (8–12 reps)

*Push-pull superset:** 3 sets/**Upright row** (8–12 reps) + 3 sets/**Decline press** (8–12 reps)

3 sets/**Pullover** (8–12 reps)

2 sets/**Crunch** (each set done until failure)

2 sets/**Reverse crunch** (each set done until failure)

Days 2 + 5 (Rest 90 seconds between sets)

4 sets/**Seated shoulder press** (8–12 reps)

2 sets/**Front raise** (8–12 reps)

2 sets/**Lateral raise** (8–12 reps)

2 sets/**Bent-over reverse raise** (8–12 reps)

*Push-pull superset:** 3 sets/**Biceps curl** (8–12 reps) + 3 sets/**Seated triceps extension** (8–12 reps)

*Push-pull superset:** 2 sets/**Hammer curl** (8–12 reps) + 2 sets/**Lying triceps press** (8–12 reps)

*Push-pull superset:** 2 sets/**Reverse curl** (8–12 reps) + 2 sets/**Triceps pushdown** (8–12 reps)

1 set/**Twisting crunch** (done until failure)

1 set/**Twisting leg thrust** (done until failure)

1 set/**V-up with a twist** (done until failure)

Days 3 + 6 (Rest 90 seconds between sets)

*Push-pull superset:** 4 sets/**Lunge** (8–12 reps) + 4 sets/**Squat** (8–12 reps)

*Push-pull superset:** 2 sets/**Reverse lunge** (8–12 reps) + 2 sets/**Front squat** (8–12 reps)

*Push-pull superset:** 2 sets/**Good morning** (8–12 reps) + 2 sets/**Side lunge** (8–12 reps)

*Push-pull superset:** 3 sets/**Leg curl** (8–12 reps) + 3 sets/**Leg extension** (8–12 reps)

Push-pull superset: 2 sets/**Standing calf raise** (8–12 reps) + 2 sets/**Seated calf raise** (8–12 reps)

1 set/**Crunch** (done until failure)

1 set/**Reverse crunch** (done until failure)

1 set/**Side raise** (done until failure)

*For supersets, do 1 set of the first exercise, then 1 set of the second. Alternate between both exercises until you've completed all your sets.

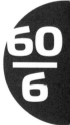

60 Minutes/6 Days a Week

Your Instant COMPLETE-BODY Plan!

Day 1 (Rest 60 seconds between sets)

3 sets/**Bench press**
(12–15 reps; 8–12 reps; 6–8 reps)

3 sets/**Incline fly**
(12–15 reps; 8–12 reps; 6–8 reps)

2 sets/**Decline press**
(8–12 reps; 6–8 reps)

3 sets/**Seated shoulder press**
(12–15 reps; 8–12 reps; 6–8 reps)

3 sets/**Lateral raise**
(12–15 reps; 8–12 reps; 6–8 reps)

3 sets/**Seated triceps extension**
(12–15 reps; 8–12 reps; 6–8 reps)

2 sets/**Triceps pushdown**
(8–12 reps; 6–8 reps)

1 set/**Crunch**
(done until failure)

1 set/**Reverse crunch**
(done until failure)

2 minutes of low-intensity cardiovascular exercise

20 minutes of medium-intensity cardio

3 minutes of low-intensity cardio

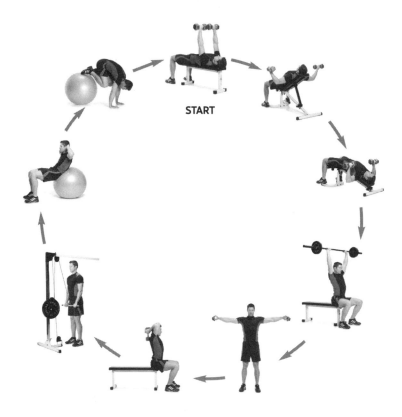

START

Day 2 (Rest 60 seconds between sets)

4 sets/**Squat**
(12–15 reps; 8–12 reps; 6–8 reps; 6–8 reps)

3 sets/**Lunge**
(12–15 reps; 8–12 reps; 6–8 reps)

3 sets/**Bent-over row**
(12–15 reps; 8–12 reps; 6–8 reps)

3 sets/**Lat pulldown**
(12–15 reps; 8–12 reps; 6–8 reps)

3 sets/**Biceps curl**
(12–15 reps; 8–12 reps; 6–8 reps)

2 sets/**Reverse curl**
(12–15 reps; 8–12 reps)

1 set/**Side raise**
(done until failure)

1 set/**V-up with a twist**
(done until failure)

2 minutes of low-intensity cardiovascular exercise

20 minutes of medium-intensity cardio

3 minutes of low-intensity cardio

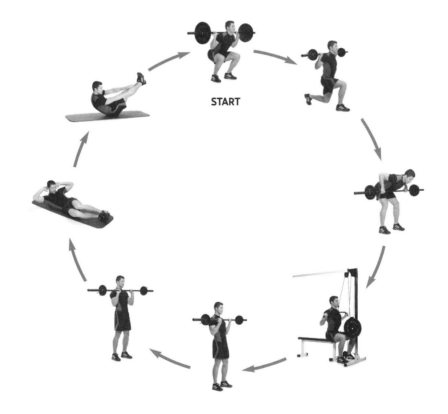

START

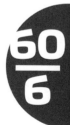

Your Instant COMPLETE-BODY Plan!—cont.

Day 3

5 minutes of low-intensity cardiovascular exercise

35 to 45 minutes of medium-/high-intensity cardio (alternate between 4 minutes at a medium intensity and 1 minute at a high intensity)

5 minutes of low-intensity cardio

Day 4 (Rest 60 seconds between sets)

4 sets/**Bench press**
(12–15 reps; 8–12 reps; 6–8 reps; 6–8 reps)

3 sets/**Incline press**
(12–15 reps; 8–12 reps; 6–8 reps)

3 sets/**Seated shoulder press**
(12–15 reps; 8–12 reps; 6–8 reps)

3 sets/**Bent-over reverse raise**
(12–15 reps; 8–12 reps; 6–8 reps)

3 sets/**Triceps pushdown**
(12–15 reps; 8–12 reps; 6–8 reps)

3 sets/**Dip**
(12–15 reps; 8–12 reps; 6–8 reps)

1 set/**Crunch**
(done until failure)

1 set/**Reverse crunch**
(done until failure)

2 minutes of low-intensity cardiovascular exercise

20 minutes of medium-intensity cardio

3 minutes of low-intensity cardio

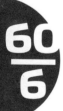

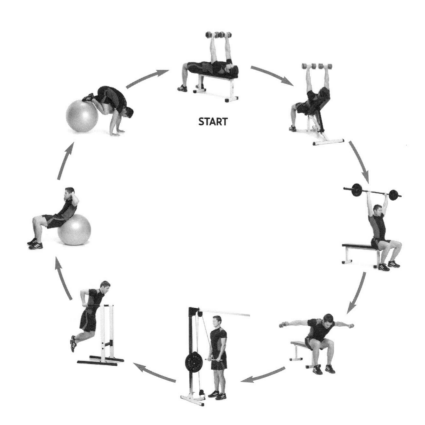

START

Day 5 (Rest 60 seconds between sets)

3 sets/**Front squat**
(12–15 reps; 8–12 reps; 6–8 reps)

3 sets/**Reverse lunge**
(12–15 reps; 8–12 reps; 6–8 reps)

3 sets/**One-arm row**
(12–15 reps; 8–12 reps; 6–8 reps)

3 sets/**Close-grip pulldown**
(12–15 reps; 8–12 reps; 6–8 reps)

3 sets/**Hammer curl**
(12–15 reps; 8–12 reps; 6–8 reps)

2 sets/**Preacher curl**
(8–12 reps; 6–8 reps)

1 set/**Side raise**
(done until failure)

1 set/**V-up with a twist**
(done until failure)

2 minutes of low-intensity cardiovascular exercise

20 minutes of medium-intensity cardio

3 minutes of low-intensity cardio

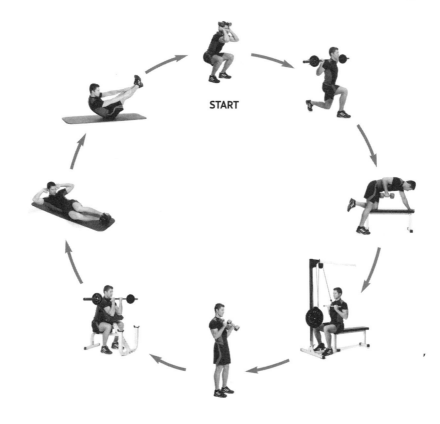

START

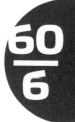

Day 6

5 minutes of low-intensity cardiovascular exercise

35 to 45 minutes of medium-intensity cardio

5 minutes of low-intensity cardio

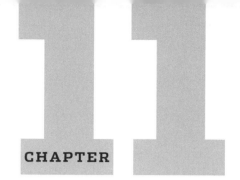
I Have 7 Days a Week

Stop right there. No one's more proud of you right now than I am for being so incredibly devoted to working out. But it's that kind of exercise eagerness that will leave you wishing you had given your body a break.

The Smart Way to Do 7 Days

Working out 7 days a week—even for the advanced exerciser—isn't the way to the fastest results, but it's the quickest way to make sure you *stop* seeing them. Your body needs at least 1 day's worth of rest, or regardless of the intensity of your workouts, you're jeopardizing your health. How? Simply put, you're compromising your immune system by overworking it beyond what it was ever meant to handle physically.

If you find yourself eager to spend your last day of the week doing something for your muscles, then make it something that treats them to the break they desperately deserve. If you're that serious about exercise, you should start taking stretching seriously, too. Letting your muscles,

tendons, and other connective tissues tighten up increases your chances of pulling them.

But if being sidelined from exercise doesn't scare you into stretching, what about the thought that you may be seeing less results for all your hard work? Maybe you don't care how flexible you are now, but forgetting to keep your muscles loose will also make them weaker in the long run. The elasticity of all your tendons, ligaments, and joints decreases over time. This can cause each of your muscles to foreshorten, and that means they'll tire out a lot faster. The good news is that regular stretching can slow down this process, so you can *always* tap into *all* the energy your muscles are capable of. Even focusing on your breathing while you stretch trains your lungs to expand as much as possible, letting you pull in more oxygen than usual for energy.

Avoiding a stretching routine also prevents your muscles from working through the most complete range of motion possible. Your muscles need to be flexible, especially during full-range movements such as squats, deadlifts, and bench presses. If you can perform an exercise through its fullest range of motion, you'll use the maximum number of muscle fibers, and that means you'll get more development within the muscles you're trying to change. On the other hand, limit that range of motion with a few tight muscles and you'll cheat your body from reaching its true potential.

YOUR MUSCLES NEED TO BE FLEXIBLE. IF YOU CAN PERFORM AN EXERCISE THROUGH ITS FULLEST RANGE OF MOTION, YOU'LL GET MORE DEVELOPMENT WITHIN THE MUSCLES YOU'RE TRYING TO CHANGE. NO MATTER WHEN YOU USE THESE 10 "ANYTIME" STRETCHES, YOU'LL ALWAYS BE HELPING TO KEEP YOUR MUSCLES FREE FROM INJURY AND FULL OF ENERGY!

Finally, pulling and tugging on your muscles can help reduce post-workout soreness. Regular stretching can increase the amount of oxygen-rich blood that your body pumps into your muscles. All this excess oxygen helps push out excess lactic acid—the leftover by-product of resistance training that causes that burning sensation in your muscles. Tack a few minutes of stretching onto the back of your workouts and you could completely dodge the next-day soreness that comes from a job well done.

Here's How to Tweak Your Week

I'm introducing you to stretching in this section, but the truth is, it doesn't matter whether you choose to exercise 1 day a week or 7 days a week. The benefits of staying flexible go beyond just giving you a respite on the seventh day of your workout.

Spending all your off-days stretching your muscles can help you get more from them when you finally return to the weights, so feel free to use any of the following routines in between your workouts. You can even opt to use each of these stretches individually whenever any muscle feels like it could use a little loosening up. (*Note:* If you're trying these routines on your off-days—and not after a workout—always be sure to warm up your muscles first, with at least 5 minutes of light aerobic activity.)

And be sure to try throwing in a shorter stretching routine at the end of your workouts. The best time to stretch is when your muscles are already warm and pliable from the excess blood that flows into them during exercise.

No matter when you use these 10 "anytime" stretches, and no matter which ones you decide to use, you'll always be helping to keep your muscles free from injury and full of energy!

The 10 Anytime Stretches

UPPER-BODY STRETCHES

STANDING CHEST STRETCH

WHAT'S IT STRETCHING? Your chest and shoulders

Stand next to the edge of a wall (or any sturdy object you can grab at shoulder level) with your right side closest to the wall. Place your right hand flat against the wall, extending your arm straight out, with your elbow unlocked. Step forward as far as you comfortably can until you feel a slight stretch along the outside of your chest. Hold for 10 seconds, then change positions and perform the stretch with your left arm.

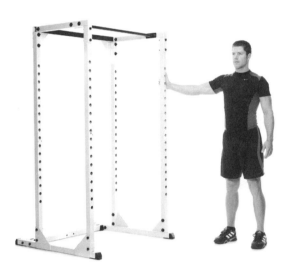 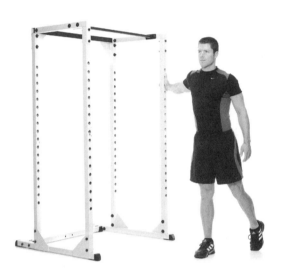

SHOULDER STRETCH

WHAT'S IT STRETCHING? Your shoulders

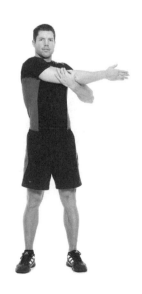

Extend your right arm straight across your chest as if you were reaching over to the left. "Hook" your left arm up and underneath your right arm, then use it to gently pull your right arm closer in toward your chest—you should feel a stretch along your right shoulder. Hold for 10 seconds, then switch positions to loosen your left shoulder.

WINGOVER

WHAT'S IT STRETCHING? Your triceps

Raise your right arm straight over your head, then bend it at the elbow so that your right hand drops behind your head. You should look as if you were about to scratch your upper back. Take your left hand, grab your right elbow with it, and gently push your right arm backward slightly for 8 to 10 seconds. Switch arms and repeat.

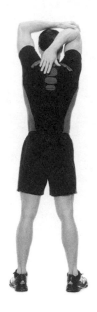

LYING SPINAL TWIST

WHAT'S IT STRETCHING? Your latissimus dorsi and erector spinae muscles

Lie flat on your back with your legs straight and your arms down at your sides. Bend your left leg and plant your left foot flat on the floor next to your butt—your left knee should point to the ceiling. Reach across your body with your right hand, and grab the outside of your left knee. Keeping your knee bent, gently pull your left leg over to your right side as you simultaneously twist your torso to the left. Hold for 10 seconds, then gently twist yourself back. Change positions—drawing your right knee up and keeping your left leg down—and repeat the stretch on that side.

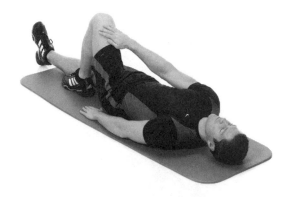
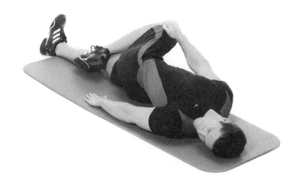

DOLPHIN

WHAT'S IT STRETCHING? Your shoulders, chest, biceps, and abdominal muscles

Sit down on the floor with your knees bent and your feet flat. Reach back as far as possible and place your hands behind you, your palms flat and your fingers pointing away from your body. Your feet should stay on the floor. Lift up your chest and arch your back so that your shoulders draw back. Tilt your head back and hold the position for 5 seconds. Relax and repeat the stretch twice more to loosen your muscles even further.

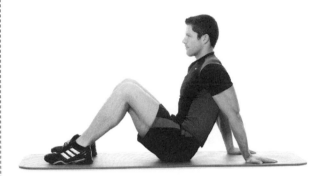 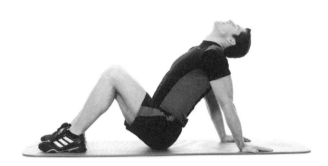

LOWER-BODY STRETCHES

TOWEL HAMSTRING STRETCH

WHAT'S IT STRETCHING? Your hips, hamstrings, and gluteal muscles

Lie with your back flat on a mat and your legs extended straight. Grab the ends of a towel with both hands and loop the center of the towel around your right foot. Keeping your head and back on the floor, slowly pull your right leg up toward you as far as is comfortable. Hold for 5 seconds, then slowly lower your leg back to the floor. Repeat the stretch once more with your right leg, then change positions to perform the stretch twice with your left leg.

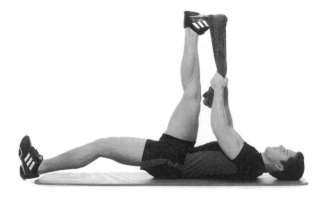

LYING QUADRICEPS STRETCH

WHAT'S IT STRETCHING? Your quadriceps

Lie on your left side with your left arm extended alongside your head and your legs straight. Rest your head on your upper arm and bend your right leg so that your right foot draws back toward your butt. Reach back with your right hand and grab your ankle, keeping your leg parallel to the floor. Maintaining this position, gently push your hip forward and hold for 5 seconds. Relax, repeat once more, then switch positions to stretch your left leg.

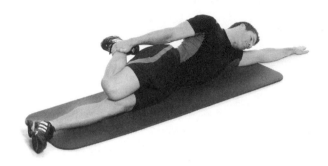

LYING GLUTE STRETCH

WHAT'S IT STRETCHING? Your gluteal muscles, your upper and lower back, and your hamstrings

Lie on your back with both legs flat on the floor. Bend your right leg and place your right foot over your leg, resting it flat on the floor on the outside of your left thigh. Grab below your right knee and gently pull it toward your chest as far as is comfortable, keeping your upper body flat on the floor, and hold for 5 seconds. Relax, repeat, then switch positions to stretch your left leg.

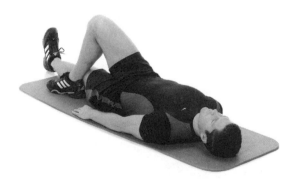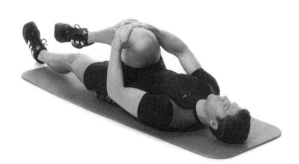

STRETCH AND REACH

WHAT'S IT STRETCHING? Your entire body

Lie flat on your back with your arms directly overhead—your upper arms alongside your ears—and your legs straight. Reach back with your fingers while simultaneously pointing with your toes. Imagine that you're being pulled apart, or that you're trying to get your hands as far away from your feet as you can. Suck in your abdominal muscles and hold the stretch for 10 seconds. Slowly return yourself to the starting position and repeat once more.

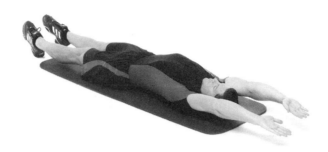

STANDING CALF STRETCH

WHAT'S IT STRETCHING? Your calf muscles

Stand with your feet shoulder width apart and your toes out pointing in front of you, then step forward with your left foot. Place your hands on top of your left thigh, just above your knee, and gently straighten your right leg until your heel is flat on the floor. Your back should be straight—hips forward—with your head up as you hold the stretch for 5 to 10 seconds. Change positions and repeat the stretch with your right leg forward and your left leg behind you.

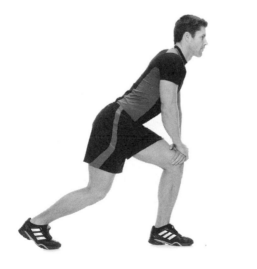
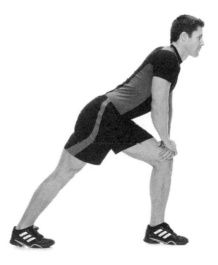

The Perfect Routines for the Time You Have

HAVE JUST 5 MINUTES TO SPARE?

Do 30 seconds of low-intensity cardiovascular exercise.

Do each of the following stretches once. Rest 15 seconds between all stretches.

Standing chest stretch

Lying spinal twist

Dolphin

Lying quadriceps stretch

Lying glute stretch

Stretch and reach

HAVE JUST 10 MINUTES TO SPARE?

Do 2 minutes of low-intensity cardiovascular exercise.

Do each of the following stretches once. Rest 15 seconds between all stretches.

Standing chest stretch

Shoulder stretch

Wingover

Lying spinal twist

Dolphin

Towel hamstring stretch

Lying quadriceps stretch

Lying glute stretch

Stretch and reach

Standing calf stretch

HAVE 15 MINUTES TO SPARE?

Do 3 minutes of low-intensity cardiovascular exercise.

Do each of the following stretches. Rest 15 seconds between all stretches.

Standing chest stretch (do twice)

Shoulder stretch (once)

Wingover (once)

Lying spinal twist (twice)

Dolphin (twice)

Towel hamstring stretch (twice)

Lying quadriceps stretch (once)

Lying glute stretch (twice)

Stretch and reach (once)

Standing calf stretch (once)

Your "FREE" Full-Body Massage!

The pros know something you may not. There's more to sports massage than just relaxing the muscles. Improving range of motion in the body, speeding up muscle recovery, preventing overuse injuries, and even softening up scar tissue from past injuries are among the running list of benefits of a good massage. It's what keeps those high-caliber athletes on the field loose and injury-free night after night.

But who has the cash for biweekly massages, or is blessed with a partner generous enough to work those knots out on call? Now you can treat yourself to a full-body sports massage anytime you want. All you need are your own two hands. It may not be as relaxing as the real thing, but self massage still helps to reduce tension, draw out the acids that cause muscle soreness, and cut your recovery time dramatically. And the fact that it's convenient and free doesn't hurt either.

HANDS

Start by gently pulling each of your fingers with the thumb and fingers of your opposite hand. Gently stroke each finger as you go, applying firm but gentle pressure to any sore or tender areas that you find. To work out the palm, loosely clasp your hands together by intertwining your fingers. Touch the thumb of your massaging hand to the

Spend Less Time . . . Complaining That You Have No Time to Stretch!

Giving your muscles the wringing out they rightfully deserve after a workout doesn't have to be the time-constraining burden most people believe it needs to be. A good stretching routine doesn't always have to be a lengthy process in order to be effective. In fact, you can loosen up almost every major muscle group throughout your upper and lower body in 1 minute. This full-body stretch may take a few steps to perform, but its yoga-based approach lets you relax your chest, back, abs, legs, shoulders, arms, and calves in seconds flat.

Step 1: To start the stretch, get down on all fours, spacing your feet and hands about shoulder width apart. Your palms should rest flat on the floor.

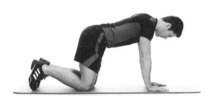

Step 2: Drop your head and slowly round your back upward as far as you can. Your hands and knees should stay on the ground throughout the movement. Hold this pose for 15 to 30 seconds, then return to step 1.

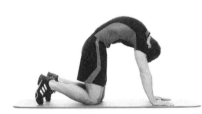

Step 3: Raise your head up so that your eyes meet the ceiling. Simultaneously lower your hips and arch your back as far as possible. You should start to feel a stretch in your abdominal muscles. Finish by

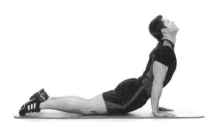

contracting your shoulder blades together to open up the chest. Hold this pose for 15 to 30 seconds, then return to step 1.

Step 4: To complete the stretch, slowly lift your butt upward, straightening your legs as far as you can without locking your knees. Your feet should end up flat on the floor with your body resembling an upside-down V. Gently lower your head down as far as is comfortable, and hold for 15 to 30 seconds.

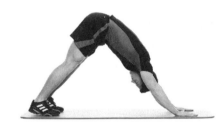

---

upper part of the sore palm (near the thumb and index finger) and apply direct pressure for several seconds. Then move your thumb around your palm in a gradually smaller spiral, applying several seconds of pressure with each spiral, until your thumb ends up in the center of your palm. Finish by stroking your thumb up and down your palm. Switch to work the opposite hand.

FEET

Sit with both legs straight out in front of you and rest one foot over the thigh of the opposite leg.

Hold your ankle with one hand and slowly rotate the foot clockwise with the other hand. Start with small circles and work up to larger circles. Then start the circle process over again in a counterclockwise direction. Repeat three times in each direction.

Next, grab your foot from the sides with both hands, placing your thumbs on the bottom and wrapping your fingers around the top. Your palms should press into the edges of your foot. Begin to stroke lengthwise up and down the foot, pressing your thumbs deep into the sole of your foot. Your fingers should apply less pressure along the top but just enough to feel a difference. Switch to making small circles with your thumbs. Don't forget to concentrate on the arch. This is where most of the tension tends to build up. Finish by gently separating and pulling on each toe, starting with the big toe, bending each toe sideways, back, and forth.

LOWER LEGS

While sitting, bend your right leg at an angle and grab the bottom of your calf muscle with both hands, thumbs behind and fingers wrapped around the front. Tilting your leg inward toward your other leg can help give you a better angle. Apply pressure with your thumbs, and slide your hands up the length of the calf muscle to the back of the knee. Repeat three times. Place your thumbs together at the top of your calf. Apply pressure and slowly pull your thumbs away from each other. (This works across the fibers of the muscle to get deeper into the muscle tissue.) Lower your hands about a half-inch and repeat this technique until your hands reach your ankle. Repeat three times. Move to the left leg and repeat the whole calf massage.

To work the shins, use the same technique of ankle-to-knee and cross-fiber strokes used for the calves, this time wrapping your hands around the front of the leg. Your thumbs should come together on the outside of your shinbone with your fingers wrapped around the calf.

QUADRICEPS

While sitting, squeeze the three middle fingers of your left hand together and press them into the top of your left thigh. Place your right hand over your left hand to help you apply more pressure. Slide your hands down your thigh until they end up just above the kneecap. Repeat the stroke, moving your hand each time to completely loosen up the muscle. Grab your thigh with both hands, your thumbs together and fingers wrapped around your leg. Begin moving your thumbs in a

circular motion as you slide your hands toward your knee. Repeat several times, then repeat on your right leg.

HAMSTRINGS

Sit on the floor with your back flat against a wall. Bend your left knee up so that your left foot is flat on the floor. This places your hamstrings in a natural and relaxed position. Make a fist with your left hand and place it behind your left knee, palm facing your hamstrings. Press in with your palm and run your fist down your left leg toward your buttocks. Repeat several times.

Lie flat on your back with your left foot over your right knee. Grab behind the back of your left knee with both hands. (Your fingers should press into the back of your leg with your thumbs on top by your kneecap.) Again, run your hands down your leg, applying pressure as you go, and repeat several times. Finally, to really work out the kinks, press the fingers of either hand into the middle of your hamstrings and slowly rub across the leg from side to side. (Apply enough pressure so that your fingers don't slide across your skin.) Move your fingers every few seconds so that you can work through the entire muscle. For all of these motions, make sure to avoid putting direct pressure on the very back of the knee. Do the same with your right leg.

LOWER BACK

Lie on your back with your knees bent, feet flat on the floor. Place a tennis ball directly under your lower back and place as much of your body weight as you can on the ball. Hold this position for a few seconds, then raise yourself up and readjust the position of the ball. Continue to lower yourself down on the ball to apply pressure to all areas of your lower back.

BICEPS, TRICEPS, AND FOREARMS

While sitting or standing, grab the inside of your left arm with your right hand so that your thumb points up toward your left shoulder. Your fingers should rest on the outside of your triceps. With your left arm straight down at your side, gently press your thumb into your biceps muscle and stroke upward toward your shoulder. Repeat several times. Place your thumb at the top of the biceps muscle where it meets the shoulder. Wrap your fingers underneath your arm so that your fingers and thumb are pointing to the left. Your right hand should look as if it's pinching the inside of your left arm. Press down gently with your thumb and push it from side to side across the tendon. Repeat several times, then continue to work the right arm. Remember to pay extra attention to your dominant arm (the one you throw or hit with).

For the triceps, wrap your right arm around yourself and cup your right hand over the back of your left arm, just below the shoulder. Your left arm should be bent at a 90-degree angle, resting across your stomach. Press your right hand into the triceps muscle and slowly move it down your arm toward the left elbow. Straighten your left arm as you go. (The area just above the elbow can be tender, so take it slow.) Your right hand should end up cupping your left elbow with your left arm straight down at your side. Bend your left arm back into a 90-degree position and repeat three times. Then switch to work your right arm.

Finish with the forearms by pressing your thumb into your forearm just above your opposite wrist. Push it up along the forearm until it rests just below the bend in your elbow, then pull it back down. To work the other side (the hairy side), press your thumb into your forearm and begin opening and closing your fist.

UPPER BACK AND CHEST

While sitting or standing, place your right hand behind your head so that your right elbow points toward the ceiling. This will keep your arm out of the way while you work on the right side of your body. Press the middle three fingers of your left hand together, bending the middle finger slightly to form a straight line across your fingertips. Now you're ready to start.

For the chest, press the fingertips of your left hand directly below your right nipple. Now gently move your hand upward toward your right shoulder, maintaining slight pressure from your hand. Once you reach your shoulder, lift your hand and place it once again below the nipple, this time a half-inch in either direction from where you originally placed it before. Repeat the process, making sure to work through the entire area of the muscle. Switch positions to work the left side.

For the upper back, press your left hand directly below your right armpit and stroke downward toward your waist. Again, once you reach the bottom, lift your hand and place it back at a different location below your right armpit. You can also go

IMPROVING RANGE OF MOTION IN THE BODY, SPEEDING UP MUSCLE RECOVERY, PREVENTING OVERUSE INJURIES, AND EVEN SOFTENING UP SCAR TISSUE FROM PAST INJURIES ARE AMONG THE RUNNING LIST OF BENEFITS OF A GOOD MASSAGE.

across the back muscle, starting from the front and moving toward the back, using short strokes as you go. Switch positions to work the left side.

SHOULDERS AND NECK

To work on your shoulders, while sitting or standing, bring your right hand across your body and place it on your left shoulder. Take your left hand and cup the bottom of your right elbow. This will keep your right hand stable when you start to massage. Bring the fingers of your right hand together and press them deep into your shoulder muscle. Slowly rock your fingers back and forth into the muscle for a few seconds, then place your fingertips a half-inch away and repeat. Continue this "press and rock" motion until you've thoroughly worked the entire shoulder muscle.

To massage the left side of your neck, place your left fingers just below your skull into the trapezius muscle. Press down and slowly drag your fingers toward your left shoulder while simultaneously tilting your head in the opposite direction away from your hand. Repeat several times, then switch arms to work the right side of your body.

CHAPTER 12

Your Minute-Man Nutrition Plan

No matter what your exercise goals, eating healthy can help you achieve them even faster. But when you barely have enough time to hit the weights, how exactly are you supposed to find time to watch what hits your plate?

The truth is, eating right actually takes less time than you think. In fact, spending a few minutes a day making the right decisions about your diet could save you from having to spend *twice* that time in the gym. That's because it typically takes less time to prepare a healthier meal than it does to work off the extra calories you would eat if you didn't spend time watching your diet.

Knowing how much time you're going to have each day to pay attention to your nutritional habits isn't always easy. Still, there is a way you can make sure you're getting the most from whatever time you have to give. What if I told you there were ways to change your daily eating habits without making major sacrifices in your diet—changes to your all-day eating schedule that you could implement anytime you wanted to?

Here they are! The following 12 tips take minutes to master, but they can take months of hard work off your schedule if you follow them each day. The three essential tips can each be done in just 4 minutes, while the other nine tips each take just 3, 2, or 1 minute—give or take—to pull off. Doing all 12 takes a total of only 30 minutes a day, yet they can give you everything you need to maintain a balanced diet.

Because this book is all about making the best of whatever time you have, all the tips are broken down by order of importance in each of the three meals: breakfast, lunch, and dinner. That way, if you have time to do only a few from each list, you'll be able to go in order and choose the most-effective dietary tips for keeping your body lean, strong, and fat-free.

My recommendation: Start with the first one at the beginning of your day, and work your way through the list. If you can't do that because of time or convenience, just pick any of them to try. Even if you do them out of order, you're still going to see results. After all, the sooner you can begin to bring these small changes into your life, the greater your chances are of sticking with them for a lifetime.

Here's your sunup-to-sunset schedule for shaving fat, building muscle, and having the all-day energy to reshape your body right now.

Sunup

THE MOST IMPORTANT THING YOU CAN DO IN 4 MINUTES FLAT!

Eat breakfast. For maximum morning energy, eat a breakfast that includes carbohydrates, protein, and a little fat. Some meals that take no time at all to make include instant oatmeal with fat-free milk and raisins; an English muffin with lean ham; a raisin bagel with low-fat cream cheese and fruit jam.

Why it's worth your body's time: Missing that first meal of the day makes you hungrier later on, which means you'll be more likely to binge and consume more calories than you truly need in later meals. It also leaves your body believing it's in starvation mode. With no food in sight, your body's nervous response is to grab whatever calories you ate the night before—and whatever you'll eat in the future—and turn it into body fat that it might need down the road. If your reason for skipping breakfast is weight loss, what you're actually doing is scaring your body into doing the exact opposite.

Blowing off breakfast can also leave you more desperate for coffee or other caffeinated beverages to wake you up, since lack of calories can leave you with less all-day energy. As you'll see later on in this chapter, the negative effects of coffee on your body can also have a huge impact on your physique. But for now, it's important to remember that the

> SPENDING A FEW MINUTES A DAY MAKING THE RIGHT DECISIONS ABOUT YOUR DIET COULD SAVE YOU FROM HAVING TO SPEND *TWICE* THAT TIME IN THE GYM.

reason you probably need coffee in the morning is because you're eating less than you should.

Opting for a meal that's a combination of proteins, carbohydrates, and fat may seem counterproductive to your weight-loss goals, but this

TIME TWEAKS!

Spend Less Time . . . Tossing, Turning, and Getting Fatter!

The closer you eat to your bedtime, the greater your odds of storing those calories as the fat you're trying to lose. That's why nutritionists recommend eating your last meal 4 hours before you sleep.

Whenever you hit the sheets, your body's functions wind down, which slows your digestion considerably compared with when you're awake. Eating a meal right before bedtime—or a couple of hours before—gives your body no choice during this metabolic slump but to turn those excess calories into body fat.

If you start feeling hungry right before you go to bed, eat a low-

calorie, low-glycemic, high-fiber food, such as spinach, cucumbers, or celery. This type of snack can curb your hunger without making your body process excess sugar, which could leave you more alert than you want to be before bed. Plus, you'll consume only a minimal number of calories from these foods, so there are fewer calories for your body to convert to fat as you sleep.

mixture is a terrific source of prolonged energy that can help curb your appetite. Your body burns complex carbohydrates as energy faster than it does proteins and fats. When you eat a meal that combines all three, it can give your body a sustained level of energy all day long. The more all-day energy you have, the less likely you'll be to reach for extra calories from other foods to provide energy later.

This rule of thumb works not only with whatever you eat for breakfast, but also with everything else you eat throughout the day. The more of a mix you can make your meals, the less inclined you'll be to reach for additional food.

HAVE ANOTHER 3 MINUTES TO SPARE?

Pour 12 glasses of water into a pitcher (roughly 96 ounces of water). Take that pitcher, stick it in the fridge, and be ready to drink from it throughout the day until you finish it.

Why it's worth your body's time: What most people don't realize is that usually, when your body's hungry, it's actually thirsty. Why is that? Because whether you're aware of it or not, your body draws a large percentage of its water from the foods you eat.

Sipping on water all day long—especially before, during, and after every meal—can leave you feeling fuller, plus it reduces your appetite during that meal and throughout the rest of the day. To stay satiated, experts agree that drinking a minimum of 8 to 10 glasses of water daily—whether or not you feel thirsty—is the standard. But going with an amount that's slightly higher than that—as recommended—is wiser, especially if you're staying physically active by using the routines in this book.

The very moment you realize that you're thirsty, your body has already lost about 4 to 5 percent of its total water. Losing a mere 1 percent of your body weight in water (roughly 32 to 64 ounces) can decrease your overall energy output by as much as 25 to 30 percent. That's because dehydration immediately puts your body in search of other sources of water within itself. Where does it find it? Your kidneys, your stomach, your colon, and—unfortunately—your muscles.

From a health standpoint, having your vital organs less hydrated makes them less effective at doing their jobs. But from a workout standpoint, having less water within your muscles leaves them much weaker during your workouts, so it's a lot harder to push them to get stronger, leaner, and larger.

HAVE ANOTHER 2 MINUTES TO SPARE?

Eat any yellow or orange fruit or vegetable.

Why it's worth your body's time: Orange- and yellow-hued fruits and vegetables offer your body multiple benefits for staying lean. Besides being a natural source of vitamins, minerals, antioxidants, and other nutrients, they tend to be water-laden and full of dietary fiber that can help curb your appetite later on.

Some fruits—such as bananas, for instance—are also loaded with potassium and magnesium, two minerals that are key for helping your muscles contract properly when you exercise. These two minerals are also responsible for preventing your muscles from seizing and cramping up later. Their color is important, since their yellowish-orange pigment means they're also filled with carotenoids—a type of phytochemical that's been shown to have an antiaging effect and to prevent certain types of cancer.

If reducing fat is your thing, then stay away from the high-sugar yellow/orange fruits and vegetables (such as pineapples, yams, corn, and carrots), and choose ones that are low-glycemic—which are foods containing carbohydrates that burn more slowly. This keeps your blood sugar low, so your body doesn't look to store fat. Some good suggestions for the few minutes you have: butternut squash, grapefruits, mangoes, nectarines, oranges, papayas, peaches, pumpkin, or any yellow pears, peppers, or tomatoes.

HAVE ANOTHER MINUTE TO SPARE?

Exchange your second cup of coffee for decaffeinated tea instead.

Why it's worth your body's time: Caffeine-rich beverages like coffee and tea wake you up by causing the release of adrenaline, a chemical that tells your body to tap into its stores of glycogen—the stored carbohydrates your body uses for energy. For that reason, it can be a smart pick-me-up for a short-term boost, but only when used sensibly.

Tossing back coffee after coffee can add a lot of unnecessary calories, depending on how you take yours. Drinking one, then switching your second and third cup of coffee for two hot cups of decaf-feinated tea can trick your body into thinking it's getting what it's used to, without adding any extra calories to your daily total.

Even if you typically drink yours black, too much coffee could still be one of the daily rituals you have that's holding your body back. Excess caffeine raises your body's production of cortisol, a stress hormone that helps your body regulate many biological functions—from controlling your blood pressure to efficiently utilizing proteins, fats, and carbohydrates. That may sound good, but for health reasons, having too much cortisol in your system can be toxic to your brain cells, leach calcium from your bones, and hinder your immune system.

Coffee can also have a huge negative impact on weight loss. Excess cortisol also kicks up insulin levels by raising your blood sugar—which causes your body to store whatever calories are left over in your system as unwanted body fat. That's why making the switch has been proven to show—in many people—an average weight loss of up to 8 pounds in just 6 weeks.

Coffee also has a diuretic effect, which means it draws water out of your body and stimulates urination. In fact, you need to drink 2 cups of water to replace the amount of liquid that a single cup of coffee causes you to lose. What makes matters worse is that many people quench that "coffee-created thirst" with even more coffee—making themselves even more water-starved during the day. Stopping this cycle before it ever starts—by drinking a hot decaffeinated beverage instead of more coffee—can ensure that your muscles are never left weaker during your workouts by dehydration.

SHAVE OFF FAT IN SECONDS FLAT . . . AT BREAKFAST!

Choose squeezed. Having juice for breakfast may seem healthy, but it's also an easy way to drink a large quantity of excess calories. To keep yourself from overdoing it, make sure you opt for juice that's loaded with pulp. You'll consume a lot more fiber than you would by drinking a glass of regular fruit juice, and that fiber can help you feel fuller throughout the day. Besides, the more pulp you've got floating in your glass, the longer it takes to drink, cutting down on the amount you would generally have.

You save: 50 calories per 8 ounces.

Choose soft. If you use butter or cream cheese, pick a brand that's whipped. Hard-packed butter and cream cheeses have more calories than their softer versions.

You save: 25 to 35 calories per ounce.

Choose spice. Instead of sprinkling sugar on your cereal or in your coffee—or reaching for a sugar substitute that's even worse for your health—try putting some cinnamon on your food. Your food will still taste as sweet, minus the extra calories that your body doesn't need.

You save: 15 calories per teaspoon.

The Middle of the Day

THE MOST IMPORTANT THING YOU CAN DO IN 4 MINUTES FLAT!

Grab three or four small snacks and save them for later.

Why it's worth your body's time: Most people break up their eating schedule into three separate

Spend Less Time . . . Wondering What's Higher in Antioxidants!

Wondering which foods to choose the next time you're looking to chow down on something healthy? Researchers at the USDA have made your job a lot easier so you never waste your body's time. Out of more than 100 different types of fruits, vegetables, berries, nuts, and spices, here are the top 20 picks, ranked according to the highest concentration of antioxidants:

1. Small red beans (dried)
2. Wild blueberries
3. Red kidney beans
4. Pinto beans
5. Blueberries (cultivated)
6. Cranberries
7. Artichokes (cooked)
8. Blackberries
9. Prunes
10. Raspberries
11. Strawberries
12. 'Red Delicious' apples
13. 'Granny Smith' apples
14. Pecans
15. Sweet cherries
16. Black plums
17. Russet potatoes (cooked)
18. Black beans (dried)
19. Plums
20. 'Gala' apples

meals: breakfast, lunch, and dinner. I've even designed this chapter to fall in that pattern. But that doesn't mean that's how you should actually eat. Whether your goal is fat loss, muscle gain, or a combination of the two, the smartest way to get your daily calories is to spread them as thin throughout the day as possible.

Eating a huge meal takes its toll on your all-day energy. Anytime you eat, your body pulls blood into your stomach to aid in digestion. The more food your body has to process, the more blood it pulls into the stomach from other areas of your body. Losing blood from your muscles and other vital organs can slow down certain metabolic functions and the distribution of energy within your system, leaving you feeling sluggish and less sharp while you digest. Larger meals also trigger an insulin surge in your system, which warns your body to desperately store body fat—not a good thing to have happen after you've just finished off a big meal loaded with calories.

Always having three snacks ready to eat between your main three meals lets you spread your daily calories out throughout your day. It may sound like you'll be eating more, but stretching out what you eat can actually cause you to eat *less*. Eating six to eight smaller meals—as opposed to three large ones—regulates your blood sugar levels so they stay even all day long. For your body, that means a constant flow of energy it can use so it doesn't have to depend on more food later on. It also leaves you feeling more satiated at your main meals, so your chances of filling up too much at lunchtime and dinnertime are even slimmer. Plus—and more important—evening out your blood sugar prevents your body from getting scared into starvation, so there's less risk of calories being stored unnecessarily as fat.

Just because I'm giving you carte blanche to snack doesn't mean I don't want you to eat healthily. When possible, choose snacks that contain a good source of lean protein (chicken, eggs, fish, or lean beef), low-glycemic carbohydrates (fruits and/or vegetables), and healthy fatty acids (such as fresh unsalted nuts). Each snack can be a mix of small portions of three different types of foods, such as two pieces of chicken breast or turkey, a cucumber and a couple of olives, or a grilled piece of tuna with a peach and a few almonds.

HAVE ANOTHER 3 MINUTES TO SPARE?

Find some beans and add them to your lunch.

Why it's worth your body's time: According to nutrition scientists at the USDA, small red beans, red kidney beans, and pinto beans were ranked (consecutively) the number one, number three, and number four most antioxidant-rich foods out of more than 100 fruits, vegetables, berries, and nuts. Small red beans had the highest concentration of disease-fighting antioxidants per serving, which experts believe helps your body to protect cells from free radicals (unstable molecules that may contribute to many health problems, including cardiovascular disease and cancer).

From a fat-burning standpoint, 1/2 cup of beans per meal delivers around 8 grams of fiber per serving. Adding that amount of fiber to any meal can instantly speed up how quickly the rest of your food moves through your body. The less time your food spends inside your stomach, the less time your body has to absorb excess calories and convert them into fat.

All that additional fiber also helps lower your risk of triggering a fat-storing insulin surge, leaves you feeling fuller so you eat less, and provides your body with a surge of saponins, a phytochemical that may reduce your body's level of bad cholesterol and prevent cancer cells from multiplying.

SHAVE OFF FAT IN SECONDS FLAT . . . AT LUNCH!

Shred it down. Having a sandwich? If you must have cheese, shredding 1½ ounces (3 tablespoons) of it can fill the same amount of space as 3 ounces of sliced cheese, cutting your calories in half. Using a stronger, sharper cheese—such as Parmesan—and then melting it can add even more flavor, so you won't need to use as much.

You save: 120 to 150 calories.

Pat it down. Having fried chicken? If you're craving something fried, try buying it the day before, wrapping it in a paper towel to absorb excess fat, then tossing it in your fridge. Chilling it first makes it easier to strip away any excess fat after it congeals. Plus, eating food at a colder temperature naturally makes you eat less, since food is more palatable when it's hot.

You save: 200 to 300 calories.

Put it down. Having pizza? Go for a slice topped with feta or goat cheese—it contains less fat and calories than regular pizza cheese. Then add at least two vegetables so that you fill up faster—and end up eating fewer slices.

You save: 200 to 250 calories.

HAVE ANOTHER 2 MINUTES TO SPARE?

Eat two pieces of a red, purple, or blue fruit or vegetable.

Why it's worth your body's time: Feel like you're having déjà vu from what you were asked to do during lunchtime? Well, the truth is, five servings of fruits and vegetables is the *absolute minimum* you should be eating every day. But this color scheme isn't about tricking you to consume at least one more for the day—even though I'd prefer you try for five—it's because switching the hue of your food can bring your body a few additional nutritional perks.

Besides being as equally abundant in vitamins and minerals as their yellow and orange cousins are, fruits and vegetables with a reddish color are also rich in lycopene, an antioxidant that has been shown to protect your body against oxidative damage as well as reduce your risk of cancer and coronary heart disease. Blue and purple fruits and vegetables, on the other hand, contain two other essential types of phytochemicals: anthocyanins and phenolics, both of which also have antioxidant and antiaging effects on your body. Picking either color—or better yet, a combination of both—will check off another necessary fruit and/or vegetable from your "must eat" list for the day.

If losing body fat is your goal, avoid red options that are high in sugar (such as watermelon, red pears, and dates), and choose one that's low-glycemic. Some suggestions for the few minutes you have: red tomatoes, red apples, red grapes, cherries, raspberries, and red peppers. On the blue and purple side, plums and raisins are higher in sugar, making the following low-glycemic choices your better bet: blackberries, eggplant, blueberries (they rank around number 60 on the USDA list—which is high—but they're also the second-highest-ranking food when it comes to antioxidants), purple cabbage, and purple grapes.

HAVE ANOTHER MINUTE TO SPARE?

Eat a handful of walnuts—about ¼ cup, or 1 ounce's worth.

Why it's worth your body's time: When it comes to your health, omega-3 fatty acids—a form of polyunsaturated fat—have been shown to boost levels of HDL ("good" cholesterol), lower the risk of heart disease by thinning the blood, and prevent various diseases. When it comes to your workouts, they also act as anti-inflammatories, giving your body relief by decreasing stiffness and swelling in your joints and muscles. But that's only if you have them in your diet, of course.

Found primarily in oily cold-water fish, such as salmon, tuna, and mackerel, omega-3s are also in certain plant-based foods, including soybeans, flaxseeds, and walnuts. The average person eats less than 1 gram of omega-3s a day. Even though there isn't a recommended daily allowance for omega-3s yet, the National Institutes of Health suggest 2 grams each day. Just 1 ounce of walnuts contains more than 2 grams of plant-based omega-3 fatty acids. That's more than you'll find in 3 ounces of salmon. So grabbing a handful of walnuts on the fly can give you your daily dose when fishing just isn't on the agenda.

If walnuts aren't your taste, try the following omega-3-rich alternatives: flaxseeds, tofu, soybeans, navy beans, winter squash, olive oil, or any cold-water fish.

Sundown

THE MOST IMPORTANT THING YOU CAN DO IN 4 MINUTES FLAT!

Eat a light soup, broth, or salad 20 to 30 minutes before you eat dinner.

Why it's worth your body's time: It sounds so clichéd to have a salad before a meal, but even if

TIME TWEAKS!

Spend Less Time . . . Preparing Your Healthy Foods!

Eating fruits, vegetables, and cereal-derived foods as close to their natural state as possible doesn't just save time, it also provides your body with even more nutrients. That's because the less processed a food is, the more vitamins and minerals it still has inside. The processing that most food goes through strips it of significant amounts of B vitamins, vitamin E, iron, and zinc. Whenever possible, opt for whole-food varieties of whatever you usually eat—you'll ensure that you get more from the healthy foods you're eating. And that way, you're covered in case you don't have much time in your day to eat healthfully.

Picking fewer overprocessed foods can also save you from having to spend more time in the gym burning fat. Heavily processed foods tend to be much higher in sugar, which causes your body's insulin level to rise and triggers the storage of excess calories as body fat.

SHAVE OFF FAT IN SECONDS FLAT . . . AT DINNER!

Subtract one step from your foods. The more un-recognizable a food is from its original self, the more heavily processed it is. For your body, that means less nutrition for your muscles and more fat for your middle. Wherever possible, try to move any processed foods you may be eating back a step, to a form closer to its original self. For example, if you like fries, eat a baked potato instead; or if you like raisins, go with grapes.

You save: 100 to 250 calories.

Divide your bad habits in quarters. Before you eliminate butter, sour cream, or dressing from your meals or switch to low-fat or fat-free versions, try using one-fourth of what you normally use instead. Fat-free versions may feel like the smarter choice, but these substitutes can give you a false feeling of safety that may cause you to eat more than you should. Devouring smaller portions of the real thing can be far more satisfying, plus it can keep you more in control of your eating habits.

You save: 50 to 100 calories.

Add some heat. Many people eat more because the flavor of their food isn't satisfying to their taste buds. To spice it up, mix something hot into your meal, such as Tabasco sauce, chile peppers, cayenne powder, or white pepper. This trick not only adds flavor so you'll be more eager to eat, but it also adds some heat, which means you'll reach for extra water in order to quench your fired-up thirst. More water means less room for calories you don't need at the end of your meal.

You save: 75 to 200 calories.

you're not dieting, this one step can be crucial to reaching your immediate exercise goals. That's because eating any type of low-glycemic food 20 to 30 minutes before you sit down to a larger meal can have a tremendous impact on what happens to the food you end up devouring.

Doing this simple trick has been scientifically proven to reduce the amount of calories you would normally consume by as much as 16 percent. That happens for several reasons. First of all, just eating something—regardless of how few calories it has—tells your brain that your body is being fed. Drinking hot water—in the form of soup—also slows down the amount of acid that's produced inside the stomach when it's empty. A combination of both of these effects can cause you to feel less hungry by the time you're ready for your dinner, so you end up eating fewer calories as a result.

No time for soup? A salad—or 4 to 6 ounces of any water-rich vegetable—works just as well. You won't get the same acid-decreasing effect as soup, but you'll be adding another source of fiber to your meal. The more fiber you have in your system during a meal, the faster that meal passes through your system, leaving your body less time to absorb calories and convert them into fat.

HAVE ANOTHER 3 MINUTES TO SPARE?

Trim whatever fat you can find off your foods.

Why it's worth your body's time: Playing surgeon by doing a little "nip and tuck" on your meat before you eat it can shave off about 20 to 25 percent of its calories—calories that serve no other purpose but to raise your LDL ("bad" cholesterol) levels, clog your arteries, and lard up the muscle you're using this book to build.

If you feel like going a step further, pick the next-healthiest cut above what you normally eat. For beef and pork, opt for cuts with less marbling—such as loin and round portions. For poultry, if you like dark meat, go with light; if you already eat light meat, then opt for the skinless variety. Or cook it by the next-healthiest method. If you prefer your fish fried, ask to have it baked or broiled. If you already have certain meats baked or broiled, then steam them instead.

HAVE ANOTHER 2 MINUTES TO SPARE?

Eat two servings of the darkest green vegetables you can find.

Why it's worth your body's time: You'll round off your day with yet another color of veggie, which, if you've followed each nutritional tip straight through the day, puts you at about the five servings that doctors recommend you eat for optimal health.

Why the mix-up of colors? Research has shown that many fruits and vegetables contain plenty of vitamins, minerals, and antioxidants that have particular cancer-fighting properties. But sticking with the same types of foods—or colors, in this case—doesn't provide you with enough of a mix of nutrients to cover all the bases. Experts agree that getting your nutrients from a *mixture* of different foods and colors helps those nutrients work as a team to keep you healthy. If you focus on just a few foods or colors, you end up missing out on certain phytochemicals and nutrients.

What's so great about green leafy vegetables? They contain vast amounts of iron, vitamin A, the antioxidants vitamin C and beta-carotene, and other carotenoids, but they're also rich in folate—one of the B vitamins that may lower colon cancer risk and maybe even heart disease risk. If you have a choice, pick the darkest versions of whichever vegetables are in the bowl—when it comes to nutrients, the deeper its color, the more nutrients it has tucked inside it. That same rule applies when you're deciding which type of vegetable to eat. Darker green foods such as spinach and broccoli contain much more vitamin C and beta-carotene than light green vegetables such as green beans and celery.

There are very few high-sugar greens (lima beans are one of the few), so feel free to pick any from this list of low-glycemic choices: asparagus, leafy greens (such as romaine, radicchio, and endive), green beans, cucumbers, spinach, peas,

CHAPTER CHEAT SHEET

Just because time is not an option in your day doesn't mean proper nutrition can't be. Here's a quick checklist so you'll always know what to reach for when minutes matter.

BREAKFAST

Have 4 minutes? Eat breakfast.
Have 3 minutes? Pour a pitcher of water—96 ounces—for the day.
Have 2 minutes? Eat any fruit or vegetable that's either yellow or orange.
Have 1 minute? Stop at one cup of coffee, or switch to decaffeinated tea.

LUNCH

Have 4 minutes? Eat three or four small snacks during the day, between meals.
Have 3 minutes? Find some beans and add them to your lunch.
Have 2 minutes? Eat two pieces of a red, purple, or blue fruit or vegetable.
Have 1 minute? Eat a handful of walnuts.

DINNER

Have 4 minutes? Eat a light soup, broth, or salad 20 to 30 minutes before dinner.
Have 3 minutes? Trim fat from your foods.
Have 2 minutes? Eat two servings of green vegetables.
Have 1 minute? Pop a multivitamin.

green cabbage, green pepper, celery, brussels sprouts, broccoli, snow peas, and zucchini.

HAVE ANOTHER MINUTE TO SPARE?

Pop a multivitamin—specifically, one that provides a minimum of 100 percent of the Recommended Dietary Allowance (RDA) for all minerals and vitamins, especially vitamin C and your Bs—thiamin, riboflavin, B_6, and B_{12}.

Why it's worth your body's time: Popping a multivitamin should never be a replacement for good

TIME TWEAKS!

Spend Less Time... Constantly Reading Food Labels to Lose Weight!

Examining the packaging of everything you snack on for its nutritional information is one way to watch what you eat, but it's not always the easiest thing to do throughout the day. Instead, taking a long, hard look at your meals from a different perspective can be just as effective for helping you lose fat and stay healthy.

If you know the answers to the following questions, you are well on your way to keeping your eating habits under control.

Do You Know What Percent of Your Weekly Meals Are Bad for You?

Most people spend their weeks eating the same meals over and over again. That means that if 60 percent of the meals you typically eat are bad for you, then there's a 60 percent chance that your next meal will be unhealthy, too. In order to get your weekly ratio, keep track of your weekly meals, checking off which ones are bad for you versus good for you. Then change your ratio by adding at least one "new" healthy meal to your weekly repertoire.

After a few months, some of the new healthier fare that you've been adding each week should stick around in your schedule, boosting your ratio of healthier meals without making you completely conscious of it.

Do You Know What 100 Calories Looks Like?

The next time you sit down to a big meal, start by splitting it up into 100-calorie chunks so that you become an expert on the actual portion sizes of everything you usually eat. After a few months, you'll start unconsciously breaking down how many calories are on your plate all the time, whether you want to or not. This can make overeating a lot harder to do, since being able to add up your meals instantly makes it impossible for many people to ignore what they're taking in.

---

nutrition. Instead, look at it as a "backup plan"—it lets your body rest easy knowing that it always has insurance whenever it's missing certain things at certain times.

Taking a daily multivitamin goes beyond just making sure your body gets enough of what it needs for functioning properly. From a fat-burning standpoint, even the slightest shortage of essential vitamins and minerals in your diet can slow down how effectively your body utilizes calories, burns fat, and provides energy.

Most people tend to pop their vitamins in the morning, but it's always better to take a multivitamin when your belly is empty, to help it absorb faster. Taking a multivitamin with your breakfast only leaves it competing against whatever

FROM A FAT-BURNING STANDPOINT, EVEN THE SLIGHTEST SHORTAGE OF ESSENTIAL VITAMINS AND MINERALS IN YOUR DIET CAN SLOW DOWN HOW EFFECTIVELY YOUR BODY UTILIZES CALORIES, BURNS FAT, AND PROVIDES ENERGY.

you've just thrown down your throat. Studies have shown that some vitamins are so tightly compressed that they are excreted before your body has enough time to draw out all the nutrients.

To maximize how your body gets those extra vitamins and minerals, take yours right before you go to bed. For even more results, try chewing it, if you don't mind the taste. Breaking it up before it hits your stomach can make it easier for your body to absorb it completely.

Index

Underscored page references indicate boxed text. **Boldface** references indicate photographs.

A

Abdominals. *See also* Obliques; Rectus
    abdominis
  anatomy and function of, 23
  exercises for
    deadlift, 60–61, **60–61**
    power clean, 96–97, **96–97**
  in 4-day-a-week exercise plan, 201
Aerobic exercise. *See* Cardiovascular
    exercise
Antioxidants, in foods, <u>311</u>, 312
Anytime exercises
  bench press, 46–47, **46–47**
  bent-over reverse raise, 48–49, **48–49**
  bent-over row, 50–51, **50–51**
  biceps curl, 52–53, **52–53**
  checklist of, <u>45</u>
  chest fly, 54–55, **54–55**
  close-grip pulldown, 56–57, **56–57**
  crunch, 58–59, **58–59**
  deadlift, 60–61, **60–61**
  decline press, 62–63, **62–63**
  dip, 64–65, **64–65**
  front raise, 66–67, **66–67**
  front squat, 68–69, **68–69**
  good morning, 70–71, **70–71**
  hammer curl, 72–73, **72–73**
  incline fly, 74–75, **74–75**
  incline press, 76–77, **76–77**
  kickback, 78–79, **78–79**
  lateral raise, 80–81, **80–81**
  lat pulldown, 82–83, **82–83**
  leg curl, 84–85, **84–85**
  leg extension, 86–87, **86–87**
  lunge, 88–89, **88–89**
  lying triceps press, 90–91, **90–91**
  one-arm row, 92–93, **92–93**
  one-arm triceps extension, 94–95,
    94–95
  power clean, 96–97, **96–97**
  preacher curl, 98–99, **98–99**
  pullover, 100–101, **100–101**
  purpose of, 43
  push press, 102–3, **102–3**
  reverse crunch, 104–5, **104–5**
  reverse curl, 106–7, **106–7**
  reverse lunge, 108–9, **108–9**
  seated calf raise, 110–11, **110–11**
  seated shoulder press, 112–13, **112–13**
  seated triceps extension, 114–15,
    114–15
  shrug, 116–17, **116–17**
  side lunge, 118–19, **118–19**

Anytime exercises (*cont.*)

  side raise, 120—21, **120—21**

  squat, 122—23, **122—23**

  standing calf raise, 124—25, **124—25**

  triceps pushdown, 126—27, **126—27**

  twisting crunch, 128—29, **128—29**

  twisting leg thrust, 130—31, **130—31**

  twisting toe touch, 132—33, **132—33**

  upright row, 134—35, **134—35**

  versions of, 43—45

  V-up with a twist, 136—37, **136—37**

  wrist curl, 138—39, **138—39**

  wrist extension, 140—41, **140—41**

Anytime stretches

  dolphin, 299, **299**

  lying glute stretch, 300, **300**

  lying quadriceps stretch, 300, **300**

  lying spinal twist, 298, **298**

  shoulder stretch, 297, **297**

  standing calf raise, 124—25,
    124—25

  standing chest stretch, 297, **297**

  stretch and reach, 301, **301**

  towel hamstring stretch, 299,
    299

  wingover, 298, **298**

B

Back. *See also* Lower-back muscles

  exercises for

    good morning, 70—71, **70—71**

    isometric, 1<u>58</u>

    one-arm row, 92—93, **92—93**

    power clean, 96—97, **96—97**

    pullover, 100—101, **100—101**

  massaging, 304, 305

Barbells

  for intermediate workouts, 29, **29**

  light, weight of, <u>44</u>

Basic eight-move exercise plan, benefits
    of, 8—10

Basics of strength training

  amount of weight, 16

  average time for completing sets,
    18—19

  breathing, 16

  looking straight ahead, 16

  pace for lifting and lowering weight,
    16—17

  paying attention to pain, 20

  repetitions, 15—16

  varying routine, 20

  warmup, 16

  workout log, 20

Beans, 312

Bench. *See* Exercise bench

Bench press, 8, 46—47, **46—47**

Bending arms and legs, correct angle for,
    <u>144</u>, **144**

Bent-over reverse raise, 48—49,
    48—49

Bent-over row, 50—51, **50—51**

Biceps

  anatomy and function of, 21—22

  exercises for

    bent-over row, 50—51, **50—51**

    biceps curl, 52—53, **52—53**

    hammer curl, 72—73, **72—73**

    isometric, 1<u>58</u>

    lat pulldown, 82—83, **82—83**

    one-arm row, 92—93, **92—93**

    power clean, 96—97, **96—97**

    preacher curl, 98—99, **98—99**

    reverse curl, 106—7, **106—7**

  massaging, 304—5

Biceps curl, 8, 52—53, **52—53**

Brachialis, 22

Brachioradialis, one-arm row for, 92—93, **92—93**

Breakfast

    benefits of, 308—9

    calorie cutting in, 310

Breathing, during strength training, 16

Butter, whipped, 310

C

Cable attachments, **30**, 31

Cable pulldown station, for intermediate workouts, **29**, 30

Caffeine, 308, 310

Calf raise

    seated, 110—11, **110—11**

    standing, 124—25, **124—25**

Calf stretch, standing, 301, **301**

Calorie burning

    from exercise, 7, 33

    in 5-day-a-week exercise plan, 229

Calves

    anatomy and function of, 26

    benefits of building, 26

    exercises for

        reverse lunge, 108—9, **108—9**

        seated calf raise, 110—11, **110—11**

        side lunge, 118—19, **118—19**

        squat, 122—23, **122—23**

        standing calf raise, 124—25, **124—25**

    split routine for, 200

Cardio machines

    for advanced workouts, 31

    when to buy, 27

Cardiovascular exercise

    activities for, 36

    benefits of, 37—38

    in 5-day-a-week exercise plan, 229

    maximum heart rate for, 34, 38—39

    for weight loss, 33, 37

    in workouts, 35, 38

Cheese, reducing calories from, 312

Chest, massaging, 305

Chest fly, 54—55, **54—55**

Chest muscles. *See also* Pectoral muscles

    anatomy and function of, 21—22

    exercises for

        bench press, 46—47, **46—47**

        chest fly, 54—55, **54—55**

        isometric, 158

        push press, 102—3, **102—3**

Chest stretch, standing, 297, **297**

Cinnamon, 310

Close-grip pulldown, 56—57, **56—57**

Coffee, 308, 310

Complete-body plan

    basics of, 35

    cardiovascular exercise in, 35, 38

    time available for

        10 minutes/1 day a week, 147, **147**

        10 minutes/2 days a week, 160, **160**

        10 minutes/3 days a week, 180—81, **180, 181**

        10 minutes/4 days a week, 203—4, **203, 204**

        10 minutes/5 days a week, 233—34, **233, 234**

        10 minutes/6 days a week, 266, **266**

        20 minutes/1 day a week, 149, **149**

        20 minutes/2 days a week, 162—63, **162, 163**

Complete-body plan (*cont.*)

time available for (*cont.*)

20 minutes/3 days a week, 183–85, 183, 184, 185

20 minutes/4 days a week, 206–9, 206, 207, 208, 209

20 minutes/5 days a week, 237–40, 237, 238, 239, 240

20 minutes/6 days a week, 269–72, 269, 270, 271, 272

30 minutes/1 day a week, 151, 151

30 minutes/2 days a week, 166–67, 166, 167

30 minutes/3 days a week, 187–89, 187, 188, 189

30 minutes/4 days a week, 212–15, 212, 213, 214, 215

30 minutes/5 days a week, 243–46, 243, 244, 245, 246

30 minutes/6 days a week, 276–79, 276, 277, 278, 279

45 minutes/1 day a week, 153, 153

45 minutes/2 days a week, 170–71, 170, 171

45 minutes/3 days a week, 192–93, 192, 193

45 minutes/4 days a week, 218–21, 218, 219, 220, 221

45 minutes/5 days a week, 249–52, 249, 250, 251, 252

45 minutes/6 days a week, 283–86, 283, 284, 285, 286

60 minutes/1 day a week, 155, 155

60 minutes/2 days a week, 174–75, 174, 175

60 minutes/3 days a week, 196–97, 196, 197

60 minutes/4 days a week, 224–27, 224, 225, 226, 227

60 minutes/5 days a week, 256–59, 256, 257, 258, 259

60 minutes/6 days a week, 290–93, 290, 291, 292, 293

Compound exercises, in basic eight-move workout, 9

Cramping, muscle, 20

Cream cheese, whipped, 310

Crunch, 8, 58–59, 58–59

reverse, 104–5, 104–5

twisting, 128–29, 128–29

Cycling, guidelines for, 36

D

Deadlift, 60–61, 60–61

Decaffeinated beverages, 310

Decline press, 62–63, 62–63

Deltoids, exercises for

bench press, 46–47, 46–47

bent-over reverse raise, 48–49, 48–49

bent-over row, 50–51, 50–51

front raise, 66–67, 66–67

lateral raise, 80–81, 80–81

seated shoulder press, 112–13, 112–13

Dinner, calorie cutting in, 314

Dip, 64–65, 64–65

Dolphin stretch, 299, 299

Dumbbells, 45

adjustable, for beginners, 27, 28

fixed-weight, for advanced workouts, 30–31, 30

hexagon, for intermediate workouts, 29, 30

light, weight of, 44

E

Eating. *See also* Nutrition plan
    nighttime, <u>308</u>
    workouts and, <u>231</u>
Elliptical trainers, 27
Energy, nutrients providing, 308—9
Equipment, exercise
    advanced
        cable attachments, **30**, 31
        fixed-weight dumbbells, 30—31,
            30
        Olympic E-Z curl bar, **30**, 31
        total cost of, 31
    basic, 27, 45
    beginner
        adjustable dumbbells, 27, **28**
        exercise bench that inclines, 28, **28**
        jump rope, 28, **28**
        mat, 28, **28**
        pullup bar, 28, **28**
        stability ball, 28, **28**
        total cost of, 28
    budget for, 27
    in gym, 26
    intermediate
        cable pulldown station, **29**, 30
        exercise bench that inclines and
            declines, 29, **29**
        hexagon dumbbells, **29**, 30
        Olympic barbell set, 29, **29**
        total cost of, 30
    location considerations for, <u>31</u>
Erector spinae, 25
    deadlift for, 60—61, **60—61**
Exercise(s). *See also* Anytime exercises;
        Cardiovascular exercise; *specific*
        exercises
    adjusted to available time, 2—3
    basic eight-move, benefits of, 8—10
    basic prescription for, 1
    for improving specific body part,
        drawbacks of, 8—9, 20—21
    isometric, <u>158</u>
    lack of results from, 2
    with longer workouts
        benefits of, 10—12
        rules for, 12—13
    obstacles to, 1—2
    small amounts of, benefits from, 5—7
Exercise bench, 27
    adjusting angle on, <u>178</u>
    for beginner workouts, 28, **28**
    for intermediate workouts, 29, **29**
Extensors, 22, 23
External obliques, 23

F

Fat, dietary
    avoiding, before workouts, <u>231</u>
    trimming, from foods, 314
Fat burning, from exercise, 7, 10, 33
Feet, massaging, 303—4
Fiber, benefits of, 312, 314
Fitness
    maintenance of, with 1 day a week of
        exercise, 143, 145
    reaching goals for, 5
5-day-a-week exercise plan
    advantages of, 229
    schedule for, 229
    time available for
        10 minutes, 232—34, **233**, **234**
        20 minutes, 235—40, **237**, **238**, **239**,
        240

5-day-a-week exercise plan *(cont.)*
    time available for *(cont.)*
        30 minutes, 241–46, **243, 244, 245, 246**
        45 minutes, 247–52, **249, 250, 251, 252**
        60 minutes, 253–59, **256, 257, 258, 259**
Flexors, 22, 23
Food labels, alternatives to reading, <u>316</u>
Forearms
    anatomy and function of, 22–23
    benefits of building, 23
    exercises for
        biceps curl, 52–53, **52–53**
        deadlift, 60–61, **60–61**
        hammer curl, 72–73, **72–73**
        power clean, 96–97, **96–97**
        reverse curl, 106–7, **106–7**
        shrug, 116–17, **116–17**
        wrist curl, 138–39, **138–39**
        wrist extension, 140–41, **140–41**
    massaging, 305
Form, importance of, 43–44
45 minutes/1 day a week exercise plan, 152–53, **153**
45 minutes/2 days a week exercise plan, 168–71, **170, 171**
45 minutes/3 days a week exercise plan, 190–93, **192, 193**
45 minutes/4 days a week exercise plan, 216–21, **218, 219, 220, 221**
45 minutes/5 days a week exercise plan, 247–52, **249, 250, 251, 252**
45 minutes/6 days a week exercise plan, 280–86, **283, 284, 285, 286**

4-day-a-week exercise plan
    advantages of, 199–200
    schedule for, 200–201
    split routine in, 199–200
    time available for
        10 minutes, 202–4, **203, 204**
        20 minutes, 205–9, **206, 207, 208, 209**
        30 minutes, 210–15, **212, 213, 214, 215**
        45 minutes, 216–21, **218, 219, 220, 221**
        60 minutes, 222–27, **224, 225, 226, 227**
Free weights
    vs. machine exercises, 34
    space needed for, <u>31</u>
Fried foods, reducing calories from, <u>312</u>
Front raise, 66–67, **66–67**
Front squat, 68–69, **68–69**
Fruits
    antioxidant-rich, <u>311</u>
    recommended, 309, 312–13

G

Gastrocnemius, 26, 200
Gluteals
    anatomy and function of, 26
    exercises for
        deadlift, 60–61, **60–61**
        front squat, 68–69, **68–69**
        good morning, 70–71, **70–71**
        leg curl, 84–85, **84–85**
        lunge, 88–89, **88–89**

reverse lunge, 108–9, **108–9**

side lunge, 118–19, **118–19**

squat, 122–23, **122–23**

Glute stretch, lying, 300, **300**

Glycogen

as energy source, 7, 10

replacing, after workout, 231

Good morning, 70–71, **70–71**

H

Hammer curl, 72–73, **72–73**

Hamstrings

anatomy and function of, 26

exercises for

deadlift, 60–61, **60–61**

good morning, 70–71, **70–71**

leg curl, 84–85, **84–85**

reverse lunge, 108–9, **108–9**

side lunge, 118–19, **118–19**

squat, 122–23, **122–23**

massaging, 304

Hands, massaging, 302–3

Head position, during workouts, 16,

157

Heads (shoulder), 21

Heart, cardiovascular exercise for,

37–38

Hexagon dumbbells, for intermediate

workouts, **29**, 30

Hip flexors, 23

Hips, power clean for, 96–97, **96–97**

Home gym, 27

equipment for (*see* Equipment,

exercise)

location considerations for, 31

Humerus, 21

Hyperextension bench, 70, **70**

I

Iliacus, 23

Iliopsoas muscle, 23

Incline fly, 74–75, **74–75**

Incline press, 76–77, **76–77**

Injury prevention

basic eight-move plan for, 10

with push-pull routines, 263

from shorter exercise routines, 6

from varying exercise routine, 20

warmup for, 16

Intensity of exercise

maximum heart rate for, 34, 38–39

measuring, with pulse, 35

Internal obliques, 23

Isometric exercises, 158

J

Joints, avoiding locking of, 144

Juice, with pulp, 310

Jump rope

for beginners, 28, **28**

guidelines for using, 36

K

Kickback, 78–79, **78–79**

L

Label reading, alternatives to, 316

Lactic acid, 17

Lateral raise, 80–81, **80–81**

Latissimus dorsi

    anatomy and function of,

        24–25

    benefits of building, 25

    exercises for

        bent-over row, 50–51, **50–51**

        close-grip pulldown, 56–57,

           56–57

        deadlift, 60–61, **60–61**

        lat pulldown, 82–83, **82–83**

        one-arm row, 92–93, **92–93**

Lat pulldown, 82–83, **82–83**

Lean-body plan

    cardiovascular exercise in, 38

    time available for

        10 minutes/1 day a week, 146

        10 minutes/2 days a week, 159

        10 minutes/3 days a week, 179

        10 minutes/4 days a week, 202

        10 minutes/5 days a week, 232

        10 minutes/6 days a week, 264

        20 minutes/1 day a week, 148

        20 minutes/2 days a week, 161

        20 minutes/3 days a week, 182

        20 minutes/4 days a week, 205

        20 minutes/5 days a week, 235

        20 minutes/6 days a week, 267

        30 minutes/1 day a week, 150

        30 minutes/2 days a week, 164

        30 minutes/3 days a week, 186

        30 minutes/4 days a week, 210

        30 minutes/5 days a week, 241

        30 minutes/6 days a week, 273

        45 minutes/1 day a week, 152

        45 minutes/2 days a week, 168

        45 minutes/3 days a week, 190

        45 minutes/4 days a week, 216

        45 minutes/5 days a week, 247

        45 minutes/6 days a week, 280

        60 minutes/1 day a week, 154

        60 minutes/2 days a week, 172

        60 minutes/3 days a week, 194

        60 minutes/4 days a week, 222

        60 minutes/5 days a week, 253

        60 minutes/6 days a week, 287

    for weight loss, basics of, 32–33

Leanness, strength, and size

    recommended repetitions for gaining,

        9, 16, 20

    rest time between sets for, 20

Leg curl, 84–85, **84–85**

Leg extension, 86–87, **86–87**

Leg massage, 304

Leg thrust, twisting, 130–31, **130–31**

Light weights, 44

Locking joints, avoiding, 144

Longer workouts

    benefits of, 10–12

    rules for, 12–13

Lower-back muscles. *See also* Back

    anatomy and function of, 25

    benefits of building, 25

Lowering weights, technique for,

    262

Lunch, calorie cutting in, 312

Lunge, 8, 88–89, **88–89**

    amount of time to perform, 17

    reverse, 108–9, **108–9**

    side, 118–19, **118–19**

Lying glute stretch, 300, **300**

Lying quadriceps stretch, 300, **300**

Lying spinal twist, 298, **298**
Lying triceps press, 90–91,
    90–91

M

Machine exercises, vs. free-weight
    exercises, 34
Maintenance of fitness, with 1
    day a week of exercise, 143,
    145
Massage
    benefits of, 302
    biceps, 304–5
    chest, 305
    foot, 303–4
    forearm, 305
    hamstrings, 304
    hand, 302–3
    lower back, 304
    lower leg, 304
    neck, 306
    quadriceps, 304
    shoulder, 305–6
    triceps, 305
    upper back, 305
Mat
    for beginner workouts, 28, **28**
    space needed for, 31
Maximum heart rate (MHR)
    calculating, 38
    for various intensities of exercise,
    34, 38–39
Meal planning, for workouts, 231
Meals. *See also* Nutrition plan
    healthy, increasing ratio of, 316

Medicine ball, light, weight of, 44
MHR. *See* Maximum heart rate
Mind-muscle connection, 201
Minute-Man Nutrition Plan. *See*
    Nutrition plan
Modifications to workouts, importance
    of, 39–41
Multijoint exercises, 9, 12
Multistation gym, space needed for, 31
Multivitamins, 315–17
Muscle groups
    back
        calves, 26
        gluteals, 26
        hamstrings, 26
        latissimus dorsi, 24–25
        locations of, **24**
        lower-back muscles, 25
        rhomboids, 24
        trapezius, 24
        triceps, 25–26
    front
        abdominals, 23
        biceps, 21–22
        chest, 21
        forearms, 22–23
        hip flexors, 23
        location of, **22**
        quadriceps, 23
        shoulders, 21
    importance of equal focus on, 21
    small vs. large
        number of exercises for working, 11,
        13, 261
        order of exercises for, 9
    targeting individual
        drawbacks of, 8–9, 20–21
        single-joint exercises for, 12

Muscle imbalances, from skipping
exercises, 165
Muscle plan
basics of, 33
time available for
10 minutes/1 day a week, 146
10 minutes/2 days a week, 159
10 minutes/3 days a week, 179
10 minutes/4 days a week, 202
10 minutes/5 days a week, 232
10 minutes/6 days a week, 265
20 minutes/1 day a week, 148
20 minutes/2 days a week, 161
20 minutes/3 days a week, 182
20 minutes/4 days a week, 205
20 minutes/5 days a week, 236
20 minutes/6 days a week,
268
30 minutes/1 day a week, 150
30 minutes/2 days a week, 165
30 minutes/3 days a week, 186
30 minutes/4 days a week, 211
30 minutes/5 days a week,
242
30 minutes/6 days a week,
275
45 minutes/1 day a week, 152
45 minutes/2 days a week, 169
45 minutes/3 days a week, 191
45 minutes/4 days a week, 217
45 minutes/5 days a week, 248
45 minutes/6 days a week, 282
60 minutes/1 day a week, 154
60 minutes/2 days a week, 173
60 minutes/3 days a week, 195
60 minutes/4 days a week, 223
60 minutes/5 days a week, 255
60 minutes/6 days a week, 289

Muscles
benefiting from shorter exercise
routines, 5–6
effects of rest on, 7, 10
opposing, push-pull method for
working, 263
rear, focus on, 158
Muscle soreness, 20
preventing, 296
Muscular endurance and leaner
look
recommended repetitions for gaining,
10, 15–16, 20
rest time between sets for, 20
Muscular size and power
recommended repetitions for gaining,
10, 15, 20
rest time between sets for, 20

N

Neck
massaging, 306
protecting, during strength training,
157
Nighttime eating, 308
Nutrition plan, 3
benefits of following, 307–8
guidelines for
avoiding caffeine, 310
eating beans, 312
eating breakfast, 308–9
eating dark green vegetables,
315
eating red, purple, or blue fruits
and vegetables, 312–13

eating soup or salad before dinner, 313–14

eating walnuts, 313

eating yellow or orange fruits and vegetables, 309

fat trimming, 314

snacking, 310–11

summary of, 315

taking a multivitamin, 315–17

water drinking, 309

O

Obliques
   exercises for
      deadlift, 60–61, **60–61**
      side raise, 120–21, **120–21**
      twisting toe touch, 132–33, **132–33**
      V-up with a twist, 136–37, **136–37**
   external and internal, 23

Olympic barbell set, for intermediate workouts, 29, **29**

Olympic E-Z curl bar, for advanced workouts, **30**, 31

Omega-3 fatty acids, 313

One-arm row, 8, 92–93, **92–93**
   amount of time to perform, 17

One-arm triceps extension, 94–95, **94–95**

1-day-a-week exercise plan
   advantages of, 143, 145
   time available for
      10 minutes, 146–47, **147**
      20 minutes, 148–49, **149**

      30 minutes, 150–51, **151**
      45 minutes, 152–53, **153**
      60 minutes, 154–55, **155**

Order of exercises, for workout effectiveness, 9

Overtraining, 13

P

Pace, during strength training, 16–17

Pain, during exercise, 20

Pectoral muscles. *See also* Chest muscles
   exercises for
      decline press, 62–63, **62–63**
      dip, 64–65, **64–65**
      incline fly, 74–75, **74–75**
      incline press, 76–77, **76–77**
      pullover, 100–101, **100–101**
   pectoralis major and minor, 21

Pizza, reducing calories from, 312

Plateaus, in exercise plan, 2, 10–11

Portion control, 314, 316

Power clean, 96–97, **96–97**

Power plan
   basics of, 33–35
   time available for
      10 minutes/1 day a week, 146
      10 minutes/2 days a week, 159
      10 minutes/3 days a week, 179
      10 minutes/4 days a week, 202
      10 minutes/5 days a week, 232
      10 minutes/6 days a week, 264
      20 minutes/1 day a week, 148
      20 minutes/2 days a week, 161

Power plan *(cont.)*

time available for *(cont.)*

20 minutes/3 days a week, 182

20 minutes/4 days a week, 205

20 minutes/5 days a week, 235

20 minutes/6 days a week, 267

30 minutes/1 day a week, 150

30 minutes/2 days a week, 164

30 minutes/3 days a week, 186

30 minutes/4 days a week, 210

30 minutes/5 days a week, 241

30 minutes/6 days a week, 274

45 minutes/1 day a week, 152

45 minutes/2 days a week, 168

45 minutes/3 days a week, 190

45 minutes/4 days a week, 217

45 minutes/5 days a week, 248

45 minutes/6 days a week, 281

60 minutes/1 day a week, 154

60 minutes/2 days a week, 172

60 minutes/3 days a week, 194

60 minutes/4 days a week, 223

60 minutes/5 days a week, 254

60 minutes/6 days a week, 288

Preacher curl, 98–99, **98–99**

Processed foods, avoiding, 313, 314

Psoas major, 23

Pullover, 100–101, **100–101**

Pullup bar, for beginners, 28, **28**

Pulse

alternative to taking, 32

desired, for exercise goals, 34

how to take, 35

as indicator of overtraining, 13

Push press, 102–3, **102–3**

Push-pull routines, in 6-day-a-week exercise plan, 263

Pushups, 47, **47**

Q

Quadriceps

anatomy and function of, 23

benefits of building, 23

exercises for

deadlift, 60–61, **60–61**

front squat, 68–69, **68–69**

leg extension, 86–87, **86–87**

lunge, 88–89, **88–89**

reverse lunge, 108–9, **108–9**

side lunge, 118–19, **118–19**

squat, 122–23, **122–23**

massaging, 304

Quadriceps stretch, lying, 300, **300**

Quality of workouts, outside factors affecting, 40

R

Radius, 21

Rear muscles, focus on, 201

Rectus abdominis, 23

exercises for

crunch, 58–59, **58–59**

reverse crunch, 104–5, **104–5**

twisting crunch, 128–29, **128–29**

twisting leg thrust, 130–31, **130–31**

twisting toe touch, 132–33, **132–33**

V-up with a twist, 136–37, **136–37**

Rectus femoris, 23

Repetitions

per set, time needed to complete, 18–19

recommended number of, 9–10, 15–16, 20

Rest

    effect of, on muscles, 7, 10

    exercise setup during, 143

    between sets, 17–18, 20

        limiting, for weight loss, 33

Results, from various workout lengths, 11

Reverse crunch, 104–5, **104–5**

Reverse curl, 106–7, **106–7**

Reverse lunge, 108–9, **108–9**

Rhomboids

    anatomy and function of, 24

    one-arm row for, 92–93, **92–93**

Running, guidelines for, 36

S

Salads, predinner, 313–14

Scapula, 21

Seated calf raise, 110–11, **110–11**

Seated exercises, advantages of, 37

Seated shoulder press, 8, 112–13, **112–13**

Seated triceps extension, 114–15, **114–15**

Serratus anterior muscles, chest fly for, 54–55, **54–55**

Sets

    intensity vs. number of, 7

    recommended number of, 9

    resting time between, 17–18

    time needed to complete, 17, 18–19

Setup for exercises, during rest time, 143

7 days a week exercise plan

    drawbacks of, 295

    importance of stretching in, 295–96

        (see also Stretching)

Shoulder press, seated, 8, 112–13, **112–13**

Shoulders

    anatomy and function of, 21

    benefits of building, 21

    exercises for

        chest fly, 54–55, **54–55**

        decline press, 62–63, **62–63**

        power clean, 96–97, **96–97**

        push press, 102–3, **102–3**

        upright row, 134–35, **134–35**

    massaging, 305–6

    split routine for, 199–200

Shoulder stretch, 297, **297**

Shrug, 116–17, **116–17**

Side lunge, 118–19, **118–19**

Side raise, 120–21, **120–21**

Single-joint exercises, 12

Single-station gym, space needed for, 31

6 days a week exercise plan

    guidelines for, 261

    for intermediate and advanced exercisers, 261

    schedule for, 261–63

    time available for

        10 minutes, 264–66, **266**

        20 minutes, 267–72, **269, 270, 271, 272**

        30 minutes, 273–79, **276, 277, 278, 279**

        45 minutes, 280–86, **283, 284, 285, 286**

6 days a week exercise plan *(cont.)*

time available for *(cont.)*

60 minutes, 287—93, **290, 291, 292, 293**

60 minutes/1 day a week exercise plan, 154—55, **155**

60 minutes/2 days a week exercise plan, 172—75, **174, 175**

60 minutes/3 days a week exercise plan, 194—97, **196, 197**

60 minutes/4 days a week exercise plan, 222—27, **224, 225, 226, 227**

60 minutes/5 days a week exercise plan, 253—59, **256, 257, 258, 259**

60 minutes/6 days a week exercise plan, 287—93, **290, 291, 292, 293**

Skipping exercises, problems with, <u>165</u>

Snacks, 310—11

Soleus, 26, 200

Soreness, 20, 296

Soup, predinner, 314

Spicy foods, <u>314</u>

Spinal twist, lying, 298, **298**

Split routine, 12, 199—200, 230

Squat, 8, 122—23, **122—23**

front, 68—69, **68—69**

Stability ball, for beginners, 28, **28**

Stairclimber, 31, <u>31</u>

Standing calf raise, 124—25, **124—25**

Standing calf stretch, 301, **301**

Standing chest stretch, 297, **297**

Stationary bike, space needed for, <u>31</u>

Steroids, 13

Stretch and reach, 301, **301**

Stretching

benefits of, 295—96

best time for, 296

in 5-day-a-week exercise plan, 229

full-body, <u>303</u>, **303**

for lower body

lying glute stretch, 300, **300**

lying quadriceps stretch, 300, **300**

standing calf stretch, 301, **301**

stretch and reach, 301, **301**

towel hamstring stretch, 299, **299**

in spare minutes, 302

for upper body

dolphin, 299, **299**

lying spinal twist, 298, **298**

shoulder stretch, 297, **297**

standing chest stretch, 297, **297**

wingover, 298, **298**

Sugar, cinnamon replacing, <u>310</u>

Super slow technique for lifting, <u>200</u>, <u>211</u>

Swimming, guidelines for, <u>36</u>

T

Tea, decaffeinated, 310

10 minutes/1 day a week exercise plan, 146—47, **147**

10 minutes/2 days a week exercise plan, 159—60, **160**

10 minutes/3 days a week exercise plan, 179—81, **180, 181**

10 minutes/4 days a week exercise plan, 202—4, **203, 204**

10 minutes/5 days a week exercise
plan, 232−34, **233, 234**

10 minutes/6 days a week exercise
plan, 264−66, **266**

Thighs. *See also* Hamstrings;
Quadriceps
exercises for
power clean, 96−97, **96−97**
push press, 102−3, **102−3**

30 minutes/1 day a week exercise
plan, 150−51, **151**

30 minutes/2 days a week exercise
plan, 164−67, **166, 167**

30 minutes/3 days a week exercise
plan, 186−89, **187, 188, 189**

30 minutes/4 days a week exercise
plan, 210−15, **212, 213, 214,
215**

30 minutes/5 days a week exercise
plan, 241−46, **243, 244, 245,
246**

30 minutes/6 days a week exercise
plan, 273−79, **276, 277, 278,
279**

3-day-a-week exercise plan
advantages of, 177−78
rules for, 178
time available for
10 minutes, 179−81, **180, 181**
20 minutes, 182−85, **183, 184,
185**
30 minutes, 186−89, **187, 188,
189**
45 minutes, 190−93, **192, 193**
60 minutes, 194−97, **196, 197**

Toe touch, twisting, 132−33,
132−33

Towel hamstring stretch, 299, **299**

Transverse abdominis, 23

Trapezius
anatomy and function of, 24
exercises for
bent-over reverse raise, 48−49,
48−49
bent-over row, 50−51,
50−51
deadlift, 60−61, **60−61**
lateral raise, 80−81, **80−81**
lat pulldown, 82−83, **82−83**
one-arm row, 92−93, **92−93**
power clean, 96−97, **96−97**
shrug, 116−17, **116−17**
upright row, 134−35, **134−35**

Treadmill, 27, 31, <u>31</u>

Triceps
anatomy and function of, 25
benefits of building, 26
exercises for
bench press, 46−47, **46−47**
decline press, 62−63, **62−63**
dip, 64−65, **64−65**
isometric, <u>158</u>
kickback, 78−79, **78−79**
lying triceps press, 90−91,
90−91
one-arm triceps extension,
94−95, **94−95**
pullover, 100−101, **100−101**
push press, 102−3, **102−3**
seated shoulder press, 112−13,
112−13
seated triceps extension, 114−15,
114−15
triceps pushdown, 126−27,
126−27
massaging, 305

Triceps extension
   one-arm, 94–95, **94–95**
   seated, 8, 114–15, **114–15**
Triceps press, lying, 90–91, **90–91**
Triceps pushdown, 126–27, **126–27**
20 minutes/1 day a week exercise plan,
      148–49, **149**
20 minutes/2 days a week exercise
      plan, 161–63, **162, 163**
20 minutes/3 days a week exercise
      plan, 182–85, **183, 184, 185**
20 minutes/4 days a week exercise
      plan, 205–9, **206, 207, 208, 209**
20 minutes/5 days a week exercise
      plan, 235–40, **237, 238, 239, 240**
20 minutes/6 days a week exercise
      plan, 267–72, **269, 270, 271, 272**
Twisting crunch, 128–29, **128–29**
Twisting leg thrust, 130–31,
      130–31
Twisting toe touch, 132–33,
      132–33
2-day-a-week exercise plan
   advantages of, 157
   rules for, 158
   time available for
      10 minutes, 159–60, **160**
      20 minutes, 161–63, **162, 163**
      30 minutes, 164–67, **166, 167**
      45 minutes, 168–71, **170, 171**
      60 minutes, 172–75, **174, 175**

U

Ulna, 22, 25
Upright row, 134–35, **134–35**

V

Vastus intermedius, 23
Vastus lateralis, 23
Vastus medialis, 23
Vegetables
   antioxidant-rich, <u>311</u>
   recommended, 309, 312–13,
      315
V-up with a twist, 136–37,
      136–37

W

Walking, guidelines for, <u>36</u>
Walnuts, 313
Warmup, before strength training,
      16
Water drinking
   importance of, 309
   with spicy foods, <u>314</u>
Weight loss
   cardiovascular exercise for, 33, 37
   lean-body plan for (*see* Lean-body
      plan)
Weights
   choosing, 16
   free, space needed for, <u>31</u>
   light, <u>44</u>
   technique for lowering, <u>262</u>
   when to increase, 16
Whole foods, benefits of, <u>313</u>
Wingover, 298, **298**
Workouts
   eating and, <u>231</u>
   expected results from, <u>11</u>

factors affecting quality of, 40

fine-tuning, 37

gauging intensity of, 32

head position during, 16, 157

modifying, importance of, 6, 20,
    39–41

recording details of, 20

types of (*see* Complete-body plan;
    Lean-body plan; Muscle plan;
    Power plan)

Wrist curl, 138–39, **138–39**

Wrist extension, 140–41, **140–41**

Wrist position, correct, 145

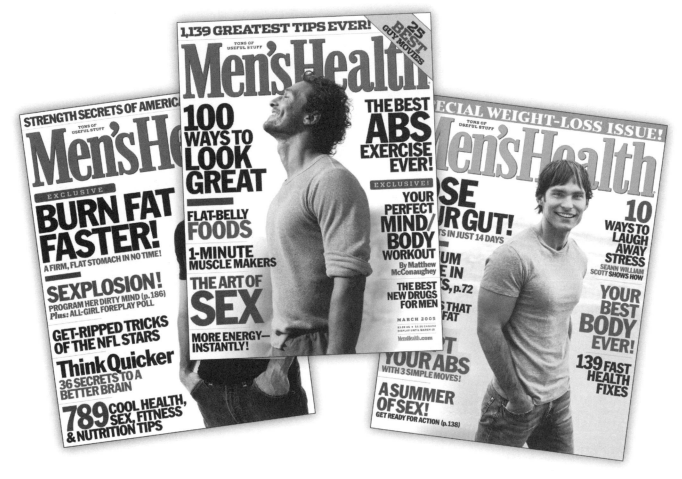

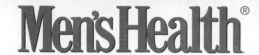
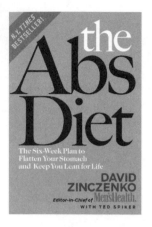
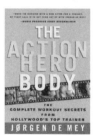
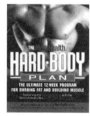
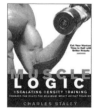
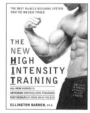
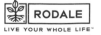